NINJA FOODI

GRILL COOKBOOK

*QUICK, EASY & DELICIOUS RECIPES FOR YOUR
NEW NINJA AIR FRYER AND INDOOR GRILL*

BY SOPHIA LEE

TABLE OF CONTENTS

VEGETABLES & SIDES............53

DESSERTS...........................65

CONCLUSION.........................76

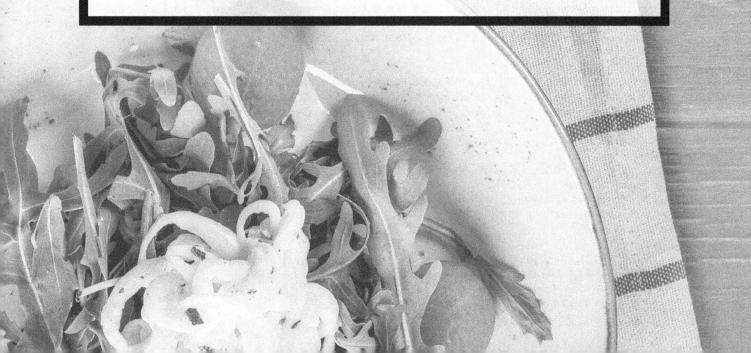

CHAPTER 1
INTRODUCTION

INTRODUCING THE NINJA FOODI GRILL

The familiar smell of burning charcoal lingers in the air as you socialize with family and friends - feasting on juicy, barbecued hamburgers, charred corn-on-the-cob slathered in melted butter, sticky chicken kebab skewers and all of the other popular "eat-with-your-hands-only" grilled delights that you have come to know well at an all-American event, namely, the barbecue. As the sun sets, you pop open your favorite ice-cold beverage and chink a cheers while coupling it with the searing steaks and browned asparagus coming fresh off the hot grill. From backyard cookouts to large scale block parties to warm evenings filled with outdoor fires, grilling has constantly been thought of as a summertime activity only. But what happens if it's not the pleasantly warm summer season? What if the weather conditions are not willing to cooperate with our best bbq wishes? Or what happens if there's no space for an outdoor barbecue grill at all?

Introducing the Ninja Foodi Grill, the grill that sizzles, sears and air fries and more.

The Ninja Foodi Grill provides a brand-new method of grilling by incorporating superheated cyclonic air that you may have heard of the original Foodi Pressure Cooker, along with Ninja's cutting edge high-density, ceramic coated Grill Grate.
Not only does the Ninja Food Grill grill foods amazingly, but it also performs a variety of other functions to make it more than worthy of adding to your collection of kitchen appliances. If you're currently thinking, "Do I really need another kitchen gadget?" let me be the first to tell you, the answer is a resounding YES. Keep reading to see to see why this one is different to all the others.

The new Foodi Grill allows for grilling, searing sizzling and, air fry your favorite foods – all with same smoky flavor of outdoor barbecuing that we all love so much, but this time from the comfort of your own kitchen. On top of that, you also get the flexibility of a Ninja Foodi, so you can additionally Air Crisp, Bake, Roast, as well as Dehydrate. I'm thrilled to lead you through your journey with the Foodi Grill - as a chef and food developer, but also as another avid Ninja Foodi user! So, let's get started with the ultimate newbie's guide on this exciting cooking adventure!

10 REASONS YOU WILL LOVE YOUR FOODI GRILL

There a more than just a few reasons as to why the Ninja Foodi Grill is a superior kitchen appliance when comparing it to other popular ones on the market. Here's what makes it so special:

Cyclonic Grilling Technology
What sets the Ninja Foodi Grill apart from any other indoor grill is the Cyclonic Cooking Technology, which incorporates an one-of-a-kind, high-density Grill Grate as well as super-heated cyclonic air that flows quickly around your food. This means you are searing your food to develop a scrumptious, caramelized char, while the air cooks your food equally from all sides rendering the fat and producing a crunchy, crispy crust at the same time. This brings the fired-up flavors, the char-grilled-ness, and the searing juiciness you would usually get from your barbecue grill-- straight into to your kitchen with ease.

No-Flip Grilling
Since the Foodi Grill distributes air around your food to uniformly cook all sides, oftentimes, you don't even need to turn or flip it to get excellent results from top to bottom. This means that gone are the days of checking and guesstimating when to flip your food that's busy cooking. Visualize flawlessly grilled fish that doesn't crumble since it's cooked evenly on all sides. With No-Flip Cooking, you get the best best char marks on one side as well as a gorgeous sear on the other. Simply set your timer, leave, and allow the Foodi ™ Grill cook your meal to perfection.

From Frozen to Char-Grilled Glory
At last, an appliance that can cook your food right from the fridge freezer! No need to wait around for it to thaw out, ever. Simply follow the Grilling Chart (link is in this book). Whether you purchased quick-frozen fish at the market or grabbed some turkey breasts from the freezer, with the Foodi Grill you are just minutes away from a tasty dinner cooked in no time.

Go Beyond Grilling
The Ninja Foodi Grill does far more than just grill. It has the ability to Air Crisp, Bake, Roast, and also Dehydrate-- all in one! Air Crisp crunchy, crispy foods utilizing little or no oil for guilt-free deep-fried faves. Transform your Foodi Grill into a stove to bake as well as roast your favorite dishes in much less time than you would usually spend. Some versions can even dehydrate meats, veggies, and also fruits to make delightful savory and sweet homemade snacky treats.

Grill Grate
The one-of-a-kind Grill Grate was crafted to quickly heat up to over 500 ° F while concurrently circulating super-heated air. This enables you to produce beautiful char marks on one side as well as sear the opposite sides at the same time. The Ninja Foodi Grill keeps accurate track of the Grill Grate's temperature level to guarantee} even cooking while reducing smoke significantly. An added bonus is that the Grill Grate is ceramic-coated for incredibly easy clean-up. Always make use of silicone or wooden utensils so that you don't damage the Grill Grate's coating.

The Crisper Basket
The Crisper Basket was created so each bite comes out flawlessly golden brown and crispy. Air Crisped crunchy French fries to go with your hamburgers or crispy brown Brussels sprouts to serve along with your juicy-yet-crispy grilled chicken is now child's play. You can additionally use the dehydrate function to create all kinds of vegetable chips and beef jerky. Just Like the Grill Grate, the Crisper Basket is ceramic coated, making cleaning simple – I know I sound like a broken record but make sure you are using those silicone or wooden utensils – you do not want to scratch this bad boy!

The Cooking Pot
The Foodi Grill's ceramic coated Cooking Pot always needs to be installed when you are using it. Whilst making use of the pot with the various accessories that come in the box (such as the Grill Grate or Crisper Basket), make sure to clean both accessories thoroughly, as oils and fat can (and do) drip down right into the Cooking Pot during usage. Once again - make sure to use silicone/wooden – I'm sure you know why by now.

The Hood

Similar to an outdoor grill, the Foodi Grill includes a special engineered hood that has a convection fan that distributes hot air to cook ingredients from all directions simultaneously. So, while your food cooks straight on the ultra-hot Grill Grate, the hot air is preserved and circulates throughout the Foodi cavity. It also captures any rogue smoke, vapors, and flavors - all of which add to bringing the outdoor barbecuing experience inside the house. Plus, the hood rapidly adjusts with the fan as well as the internal temperature levels, so you are able to Air Crisp, Bake, Roast, and also Dehydrate with this one device. The powerful fan unleashes ultra-hot air around your food to crisp and caramelizes it, but it can swiftly adjust itself to slower speeds and reduced temperatures to dehydrate fruits, veggies and meat for delicious sugar-free snacks.

The Splatter Guard

Situated on the underside of the hood, the splatter shield keeps the ultra-hot heating element clean and protects against smoke circulating. It is completely removable (for cleaning purposes only) but always ensure that it remains in place when the unit is on and cooking – it's an important piece of the cooking process!

The Grease Collector

The grease collector sits at the rear of the device to ensure that any kind of grease or oils that get trapped by the hood does not make its way to your kitchen counter. Although you'll commonly find the collector totally empty, I would suggest inspecting it after each usage.

KEY FUNCTIONS OF YOUR NEW FOODI GRILL

Now that you know how the parts of the Foodi Grill operate, its time to dive into the all-important functions. Below I outline the five main types of cooking you are able to do in your Foodi Grill After reading this chapter you will soon realize that it's just so much more than just a grill! I also give you a rundown on how to use each function, why it is unique from standard functions of similar appliances, and the variety of foods you canlook forward to making.

Grill

At its core, the Foodi Grill is a professional indoor grill. To unlock a swathe of grilling possibilities, use of the various grill control settings is key. Each different setting is specifically designed for various types of food. Put your Cooking Pot and Grill Grate in the Foodi, then let it preheat completely before adding your food for best results. To start using the Grill function, first select the Grill Grate temperature setting and use the below guide:

Low – Best for bacon, sausages and calzones. Try cooking your breakfast sides on the grill versus the span or skillet to keep your kitchen completely smoke free and your guests impressed.

Medium – Best for frozen and marinated meats of all kinds.

High – Best for proteins such as steaks, chicken, hot dogs and hamburgers.

Max – Best for grilled veggies, fruit, fresh and frozen seafoods, kebabs and glorious pizza.

Air Crisp

With the Air Crisper function, you can achieve that mouthwateringly crispy, crunchy, golden brown texture without all the unhealthy fats and oils that usually come with it. Using the simple Air Crisp feature in conjunction with the Crisper Basket to cook your all-time favorite food like thin cut fries, onion rings, or even chicken nuggets- from the freezer straight into the Foodi. Air Crisp is also great for fresh vegetables, like Brussels sprouts. Make sure that you shake the Basket or move the food around once or twice to ensure the crispiest, most evenly cooked results. Everyone's preferences differ, so don't be afraid of sneeking-a-peek under the Crisping Lid every now and then. This way you know exactly when to remove your food – once it's crisped to your exact liking.

Bake

If that wasn't enough Foodi Grill also performs just a as a mini convection oven would, if not better. The only thing you need is the Cooking Pot and a cake tin to bake fresh breads, delicious cakes, homemade pies, sweet treats, and more - in far less time than your oven could. To top it off it preheats in less than 3 minutes – dessert for the first course anyone?

Roast

The Foodi Grill would not be complete without a Roast function. You can make everything from a falling-of-the-bone, slow-roasted pot roast to some savory appetizers and sides. Just place large pieces of your protein directly In the Cooking Pot and hit the Roast function - the rest is magic.

Dehydrate

Dehydrators can be expensive, take up tons of space in the kitchen. With the Foodi™ Grill, you can dehydrate fruits, vegetables, meats, herbs, and more without adding another appliance to your collection.

Now that we understand all the basics of the Ninja Foodi Grill, it's time for the fun part: FOOD! Get your apron ready and let's get cooking!

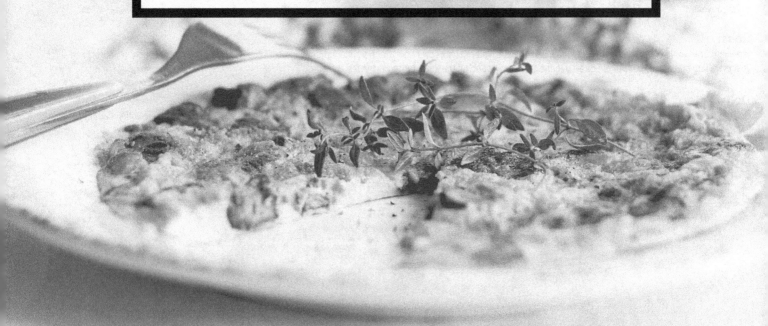

CHAPTER 2

BREAKFASTS

CHEESY POTATO OMELET WITH PEPPERS

PREP TIME: 15 MINS | COOK TIME: 35 MINS | SERVES 2

INGREDIENTS:

- 1/8 tsp. Sea salt
- 1/8 tsp. White pepper
- 1 ¾ tbsp. Canola oil
- 6 Eggs (medium, gently beaten)
- 2.63 oz. (5 1/3 tbsp. approx.) Cheddar (shredded)
- 1 tbsp. Parmesan (fresh, shredded)

- 2 Potatoes (boiled halfway, diced)
- 1 Onion (chopped)
- ½ Red bell pepper (de-seeded, diced)
- 3.5 oz. cup Button mushrooms (quartered)
- 3.5 oz. cup Baby tomatoes (halved)
- Fresh oregano for garnish (chopped)

DIRECTIONS:

1. Gently beat the eggs, pepper, and salt in a medium-sized bowl. Add cheddar and parmesan cheese to the egg mixture and fold until the ingredients combine well. Remember to leave some cheddar and parmesan to sprinkle on top of the omelet later.
2. Place the cooking pot inside the grill, and secure the hood. Choose the 'GRILL' option and set the timer for 20 minutes at LOW temperature. Press the START/STOP button to start the preheating process.
3. When you hear the unit beep, open the hood, and add the canola oil to the cooking pot. Wait for it to heat. Once the oil is ready, add the chopped onions and close the hood. Allow the onions to cook for 5-7 minutes while stirring at regular intervals. Continue cooking the onions until they wilt and turn translucent.
4. Add peppers to the cooking pot and close the hood. Cook the pepper for 3 minutes or until they soften. Next, add mushrooms and diced potatoes to the cooking pot and cook for another 4 minutes. Make sure to keep stirring the vegetables regularly.
5. Add the egg mixture, and evenly spread the mixture around the pot.
6. Wait for the egg to set a little, and then add the sliced tomatoes. Secure the grill hood and cook for 3-4 minutes or until the cheese starts to turn brown.
7. Add a generous dash of chopped oregano and cheese on top of the omelet, and allow it to cook for another minute. Press the START/STOP to turn the grill off.
8. Use thick oven mitts or gloves to lift the pan from the Ninja Foodi grill. Use a soft silicone spatula to make sure the sides of the omelet are free, and then gently tilt the pot to tip the omelet onto a serving plate. Cover the plate with another adequately sized dish and turn it 180° to make sure the cheesy side is facing up.
9. Slice the omelet as preferred and serve warm.

GRILLED GERMAN PANCAKES

PREP TIME: 10 MINS | COOK TIME: 20 MINS | SERVES 3

INGREDIENTS:

- 4 Eggs (Separate the yolks from the whites)
- 1/4 tsp. Salt
- 2.45 oz. Caster sugar (or white granulated sugar)
- 5.25 oz. Plain flour (or any preferred flour)
- 8.75 oz. Quark

- 0.35 oz. (6 tsp. approx.) Butter
- 3.5 oz. Milk

DIRECTIONS:

1. In a large-sized bowl, beat the egg whites until stiff peaks form. Set the bowl aside.
2. Place the cooking pot (without the grill plate) and secure the hood. Choose the 'GRILL' option and set the timer for 8 minutes at HIGH temperature. Press the START/STOP button to commence the preheating process.
3. In a medium-sized bowl, add the sugar, salt, quark, egg yolks, and milk. Stir the mixture until the ingredients are well blended. Next, add in the flour and egg whites and proceed to fold the batter gently.
4. Once the unit beeps and is ready to cook, open the hood to add butter to the cooking pot. Once the butter has melted, pour the batter and spread it evenly across the pot's surface. Secure the lid once again, and cook the pancake batter for 8 minutes.
5. Once the cooking cycle is complete, check if the pancake is evenly cooked and light brown. Cut the pancake into bite-sized pieces with the help of a silicone spatula.
6. Transfer the grilled German pancake to a serving plate, and serve warm with preferred syrup or preserve.

GOLDEN CHEESE SCONES WITH CHIVES

PREP TIME: 5 MINS | COOK TIME: 35 MINS | SERVES 4

INGREDIENTS:

- 1/2 tsp. Salt
- 1 1/4 tsp. Baking powder
- 1 Egg
- 3.5 oz. (7 tbsp. approx.) Butter (softened)
- 4 tbsp Crème Fraiche
- 1.4 oz. (2 2/3 tbsp. approx.) Mature cheddar (shredded)

- 9.5 oz. Plain flour
- 1 tbsp. Chives (minced)

Brushing
- 1 Egg
- 1 tbsp. Milk

DIRECTIONS:

1. Add baking powder, salt, flour, cheddar, and chives in a large-sized bowl and mix well. Proceed to add softened butter, crème fraiche, egg, and combine the ingredients until a batter forms. Place the mixture on a clean work surface and knead until a dough forms. Be careful about not kneading the dough too much, as this can affect the texture of the scones.
2. Place the cooking pot inside the Foodi Grill and secure the hood. Set the timer for 17 minutes at 338°F and press the START/STOP button to start preheating the grill.
3. Roll out the dough to a 3-cm thickness on the work surface. Next, cut out the scones with the help of a biscuit cutter. Collect the leftover dough, and repeat the process until all the dough has been used up.
4. Add the brushing ingredients in a small-sized bowl. Gently beat to mix the ingredients and touch up the tops of the scones using the brushing mixture.
5. When you hear the unit beep, open the grill hood and spray an even coat of cooking spray on the cooking pot to grease it. Add the scones and secure the lid. Allow the scones to cook for the duration of the required time.
6. Once the cooking cycle is over, transfer the scones to a serving plate and allow them to cool. You can serve the scone with jam, butter, chutney, etc.

CREAMY PORK & ASPARAGUS FRITTATA

PREP TIME: 10 MINS | COOK TIME: 30 MINS | SERVES 4

INGREDIENTS:

- 8 oz. Heavy cream
- 8 Eggs
- 1 cup Cheddar (shredded)
- ½ tsp. Salt
- ¼ tsp. Black Pepper

- 1 tsp. Onion powder
- ½ bunch Asparagus
- 1 Red Pepper (sliced)
- ½ lb. Pork sausage
- Butter to grease the pan

DIRECTIONS:

1. Place the grill grate inside the unit and close the grill hood. Choose the 'GRILL' option, and set the timer for 8 minutes at 'MAX' temperature. Press the START/STOP button to initiate preheating.
2. The Foodi grill will be ready for cooking once it beeps. Open the hood, and place the asparagus, red pepper, and sausages on the grill grate.
3. Secure the hood and cook for at least 4 minutes. Next, open the lid to the vegetables and the sausages. Close the hood and proceed to cook for the remainder of the time.
4. Shift the grilled vegetables and sausages to a plate. Take the grill grate out of the unit.
5. In a bowl, whisk the cream, onion powder, salt, black pepper, and eggs until mixed well.
6. Next, grease a baking pan (or the Ninja multi-purpose pan) with butter.
7. Choose the 'BAKE' option and set the timer for 20 minutes at 350°F. Press the START/STOP button for pre-heating.
8. Slice the grilled vegetables and sausages into small bite-size pieces and mix with shredded cheddar. Add this mix to the greased pan and even out with a spatula or spoon.
9. Next, pour the egg mixture over the sausages, vegetables, and cheese in the pan. Remember to even the frittata mixture.
10. Put the pan inside the Foodi grill, and cook for 20 minutes. Once the frittata is cooked, allow it cool for 5 minutes minimum before serving.

FRUITY YOGHURT WITH BAKLAVA CRUMBLE

PREP TIME: 15 MINS | COOK TIME: 25 MINS | SERVES 4

INGREDIENTS:

Yogurt Dressing
- Leftover grilled fruit glaze
- 5 oz. yogurt

Grilled Fruit
- Zest of ½ Orange
- 2 Peaches (halved or quartered)

- 1 tbsp. Water
- 1 tbsp. Honey
- 2 Plums (halved or quartered)

Baklava Crumble
- 1 pinch of Sea Salt
- 2 tsp. Cinnamon (ground)

- ½ tsp. Ginger (ground)
- 1 tsp. Cardamom (ground)
- 1/3 cup whole grain oats
- 1 ½ tbsp Sugar
- 1 ½ tbsp Walnuts (roughly chopped)
- 2 ½ tbsp. Butter

DIRECTIONS:

1. Start by placing the crisper pan into the Foodi Grill cooking pot. Use the crisper basket (by lining its base with tin foil) if you don't have the crisper pan. Pick the AIR FRY option, and set the timer for 5 minutes at 302°F. To start the preheating process, press the START/STOP button.
2. Gather the ingredients for baklava crunch while the grill is preheating. Add the ingredients in an adequately sized bowl, add butter, and proceed to mix the ingredients until it starts looking like bread crumbs.
3. After preheating, add the baklava crunch mixture to the crisper pan (or basket) and spread it out using a spatula or spoon. Place the pan inside the unit and cook for 2 1/2 minutes. Take the pan out, stir the crunch mixture, and place it back in the unit for the remaining cooking time.
4. Make the glaze by adding the orange zest, water, and honey in a bowl. Set aside.
5. Remove the crisper pan and the cooking pot from the unit once the cooking cycle is complete. Take the crisper pan out from the pot and let it cool.
6. Place the grill plate inside the cooking pot. Next, proceed to select the GRILL option, set the timer for 6 minutes at the highest temperature setting. Press the START/STOP button to initiate the pre-heating process.
7. Once the 'ADD FOOD' sign appears, proceed to glaze the fruits on the flat side. Next, place the fruit on the grill plate face down. Glaze the top of the fruits and then secure the lid.
8. After three minutes have passed, open the lid to glaze the fruit tops again. Shut the lid and wait for the remainder of the cooking time.
9. Add the yogurt to the remaining glaze mix and set aside. Once the cooking cycle is over, serve the fruit with the yogurt dressing and baklava crackle immediately.

SUMMER GRILLED PINEAPPLES & PEACHES

PREP TIME: 10 MINS | COOK TIME: 4 MINS | SERVES 4

INGREDIENTS:

- 6 tbsp. Honey (equally divided)
- 1/2 lb. Strawberries (rinsed, cored, halved)
- 2 Peaches (pitted, quartered)
- 9 oz. can of Pineapple chunks (reserve the juice)
- 1 tbsp. Lemon juice (freshly squeezed)

DIRECTIONS:

1. Place the grill grate inside the Foodi Grill, and secure the hood. Choose the 'GRILL' option and set the timer for 4 minutes at MAX temperature. Press the START/STOP button to initiate the preheating process.
2. In a large-sized bowl, combine all the fruits and 3 tbsp. of honey. Use a large spoon or toss the fruit to coat with honey.
3. Once the unit beeps, start the cooking process by arranging the fruits on the grill grate. Lightly press down on the fruits to ensure grill marks. Secure the grill hood and cook for 4 minutes.
4. Combine the remaining honey, lemon juice, and pineapple juice in an adequately-sized bowl.
5. Once the cooking cycle is complete, transfer the fruit to a large-sized bowl and toss with the honey dressing. Serve the dessert right away.

BREAKFAST STUFFED PEPPERS

PREP TIME: 10 MINS | COOK TIME: 15 MINS | SERVES 4

INGREDIENTS:

- Sea salt (as required)
- 4 Eggs (large)
- 4 Bell peppers (de-seeded, without tops)
- 4 Bacon slices (cooked, chopped)
- 1 cup Cheddar (shredded)
- Fresh parsley for garnish (chopped)

DIRECTIONS:

1. Place the crisper basket inside the Foodi grill and secure the grill hood. Choose the 'AIR CRISP' option and set the timer for 15 minutes at 390°F. To start the preheating process, start the START/STOP button.
2. Next, equally distribute the bacon and cheese among the four bell peppers. Break an egg and place one in each bell pepper. Season the bell peppers with salt.
3. Once the grill is heated and you can the beeps, carefully arrange the bell pepper inside the crisper basket. Cook for 15 minutes or until the egg whites are cooked through.
4. After the bell peppers are ready, transfer the bell peppers to a serving plate and garnish with fresh parsley.

BANANA TOAST WITH COCONUT CREAM

PREP TIME: 15 MINS | COOK TIME: 10 MINS | SERVES 4

INGREDIENTS:

- 2 Eggs (large)
- 1 ½ tsp. Vanilla extract (equally divided)
- ½ tsp. Cinnamon (ground)
- ½ tbsp. Icing Sugar
- 1 tbsp. Brown sugar (equally divided)
- ¾ cup Coconut milk (lite)
- 2 tbsp. Butter (room temperature)
- 1 cup Bananas (peeled, sliced)
- 4 Brioche bread slices
- 15 oz. can of Full-fat coconut milk (refrigerate overnight)

DIRECTIONS:

1. Open the full-fat coconut milk can from the bottom. Make sure not to shake the can. Drain away the liquid collected at the bottom of the can, and take out the thick coconut cream in a medium-sized bowl. Whip the coconut cream for 3-5 minutes or until soft peaks have formed.
2. Add the icing sugar and 1/2 tsp of vanilla extract to the coconut cream and whip again until the mixture turns creamy. Set the bowl in the refrigerator to cool.
3. Place the grill grate inside the unit and secure the hood. Choose the 'GRILL' option and set the timer for 15 minutes at MAX temperature. Press the START/STOP button to start the preheating.
4. Sprinkle the sliced bananas evenly with 1/2 tablespoon of brown sugar.
5. Whisk the lite coconut milk in a large-sized bowl with the remaining vanilla extract, cinnamon, and eggs.
6. Place the bananas on the grill grate once the unit beeps and is ready for cooking. Press down on the bananas gently to ensure grill marks. Secure the hood and cook for 4 minutes, without flipping the bananas.
7. Next, butter both sides of the bread and place one slice in the egg mixture. Allow it to soak for a minute. Turn the slice over, let it soak, and repeat the process with the remaining brioche bread slices. Once done, sprinkle one side of each toast with 1/2 tablespoon of brown sugar.
8. When 4 minutes have passed, take the bananas out from the grill and set aside. Switch the temperature setting to 'HIGH' and arrange the bread on the grill grate. Close the grill hood and cook the bread for 5-6 minutes or until golden brown. During the cooking process, keep checking the slices to ensure an even cook.
9. Take the toast out of the grill, and arrange on a serving plate. Top the slices with bananas and coconut cream.

ITALIAN SAUSAGE & PEPPERS

PREP TIME: 5 MINS | COOK TIME: 22 MINS | SERVES 4

INGREDIENTS:

- Sea salt (as required)
- Canola oil (for brushing)
- Black pepper (freshly ground, as required)
- 8 Bell peppers (mini)
- 2 Radicchio heads (cut into 12 wedges total)
- 12 Italian sausage links (hot or sweet based on preference)

DIRECTIONS:

1. Place the grill grate inside the Foodi grill and close the lid. Proceed with the 'GRILL' option and set the timer for 22 minutes at MAX temperature. Press the START/STOP button to start pre-heating.
2. Brush the Radicchio wedges and bell peppers with oil and season with salt and pepper as you wait for the preheating cycle to complete.
3. When you hear the unit beep, it's ready for grilling. Arrange the seasoned vegetables on the grill grate, place it in the unit, and secure the grill hood. Cook the vegetables for 10 minutes, and do not attempt to turn the vegetables over yet.
4. Use a fork or a knife tip to poke the Italian sausages, and then brush them with oil.
5. When 10 minutes are up, transfer the vegetables from the grill grate to a plate. Next, arrange the sausages on the grate, and set the timer for 12 minutes at LOW temperature.
6. After 6 minutes, open the hood and flip the sausages to ensure an even grill. Close the lid and cook for the remaining time.
7. Transfer the sausages and vegetables to a large serving plate and enjoy the meal.

BEEFY BREAKFAST POCKETS

PREP TIME: 15 MINS | COOK TIME: 23 MINS | SERVES 4

INGREDIENTS:

- Sea salt (as required)
- 2 tbsp. Canola oil
- Black pepper (freshly ground, as required)
- Flour (for dusting)
- 3 Eggs (large, gently beaten)
- 1 cup Cheddar (shredded)
- 1/3 Cup Scallion stalks (chopped)
- 6 oz. pack of Breakfast sausages (crumbled)
- 16 oz. pack of Pizza dough

DIRECTIONS:

1. Choose the 'ROAST' option and set the timer for 15 minutes at 375°F. To initiate the preheating cycle, press the START/STOP button.
2. Once the unit is preheated and beeps, arrange the sausages in the cooking pot. Cook for 10 minutes. Keep looking in on the sausages every two minutes, and try and break down the big pieces with a wooden utensil.
3. Once 10 minutes are up, add the bell pepper, scallions, and eggs to the cooking pot and stir until the mixture is well blended. Secure the grill hood and let the ingredients cook for the remaining time. Open the hood once or twice to stir the mixture and ensure an even cook. After the mixture is cooked through, season it with salt and pepper. Then, transfer to a medium-sized bowl and set aside to cool.
4. Place the crisper basket inside the Foodi grill and choose the 'AIR CRISP' option. Set the timer for 8 minutes at 350°F. Start the preheating process.
5. Divide the pizza dough into four equal portions, before lightly dusting a work surface with flour. Roll out each portion of dough until it's at a 5-inch thickness all around. Divide the cooked egg mixture and add an equal share on each piece of dough. Next, fold the dough over to form a semicircle, and stick the sides of the dough with water. Finally, brush the top of each pocket with oil.
6. Once the unit is preheated, transfer the beef pockets inside the crisper basket to cook. Cook the beef pockets until they're golden brown, or for 8 minutes.

SWEET & SPICY GRAPEFRUIT

PREP TIME: 5 MINS | COOK TIME: 10 MINS | SERVES 4

INGREDIENTS:

- Sea salt (as required)
- 2 Grapefruits (halved)
- 2 tbsp. Demerara Sugar (or raw cane sugar)
- 1 tsp. Cinnamon (ground)

DIRECTIONS:

1. Place the grill grate in the Ninja Foodi grill and set the timer for 7 minutes at HIGH temperature. Press the START/STOP button to start the preheating process.
2. Take the halved grapefruits and sprinkle generously with sugar. Next, spatter the cinnamon and salt on top of the fruit, and set aside.
3. Once the unit beeps and is ready to cook, open the hood, and arrange the fruit on the grate (cut-side down). Secure the grill and allow the cooking cycle to commence. Once 7 minutes are up, transfer the grilled grapefruits to a serving plate and serve.

CREMINI & CHEESE FRITTATA

PREP TIME: 10 MINS | COOK TIME: 10 MINS | SERVES 4

INGREDIENTS:

- Sea salt (as required)
- Black pepper (as required)
- 4 Eggs (large)
- ¼ cup Milk
- 4 Cremini mushrooms (sliced)
- ½ Bell pepper (de-seeded, diced)
- ½ cup Cheddar (shredded)
- ½ Onion (chopped)

DIRECTIONS:

1. Whisk the eggs and milk in a medium-sized bowl, and add black pepper, salt, onion, mushrooms, bell pepper, and cheese. Fold this mixture with a spoon until blended well.
2. Choose the 'BAKE' option and set the timer at 400°F for 10 minutes. Press the START/STOP button to start pre-heating.
3. Next, transfer the egg mixture from the bowl to an 8-inch baking pan (or the Ninja multi-purpose pan) and spread it out equally.
4. When you hear the unit beep, put the pan inside the grill, and close the grill hood. Cook the frittata for 10 minutes at least or until the frittata turns golden.

SAVORY BREAKFAST BUNDLES

PREP TIME: 35 MINS | COOK TIME: 10 MINS | SERVES 4

INGREDIENTS:

- 1/8 tsp. Salt
- 1/8 tsp. Black pepper (freshly ground)
- 4 Eggs (large)
- 2 oz. Butter (melted)
- 2 oz. Cream cheese (divided into 4 equal pieces)
- ¼ cup Provolone cheese (shredded)
- 2 tsp. Chives (finely chopped)
- 5 Phyllo sheets (14x9 in.)
- ¼ cup Ham (cooked, diced)

DIRECTIONS:

1. Set the timer on the Ninja Foodi grill for 10 minutes at 325°F. Press the START/STOP button to commence the preheating process.
2. Place one phyllo sheet on a clean work surface, brush it with butter, and place another phyllo sheet on top of it. Repeat this process until you have a stack of 5 phyllo sheets. Next, cut the stack of phyllo sheets in half crosswise and then lengthwise (horizontally and vertically). Remember to keep a damp cloth handy to cover the sheets and to keep them from frying out.
3. Next, grease four 4-oz. ramekins and place one part of the stacked phyllo sheet in each ramekin. Add one cube of cream cheese per ramekin. Then carefully break an egg in each dish, and season with salt and pepper. Add equal quantities of provolone cheese, chives, and ham. Finally, gently bring the ends of the phyllo sheets together above the filling and pinch firmly to form the bundles.
4. When the unit beeps, place the air-fryer basket inside the grill. Arrange the ramekins on the fryer basket, brush the dough with butter, and cook for 10 minutes or until the breakfast bundles turn a lovely golden brown.

TROPICAL FRENCH TOAST

PREP TIME: 10 MINS | COOK TIME: 15 MINS | SERVES 4

INGREDIENTS:

- Cooking oil or spray
- 3 Eggs (large)
- ½ tsp. Vanilla essence
- ¼ cup Sugar
- ½ cup Coconut flakes
- ¼ cup milk
- 1 cup Coconut milk
- 10 Pineapple slices (peeled, with ¼ inch thickness)
- 8 Brioche bread slices

DIRECTIONS:

1. Whisk the vanilla essence, eggs, milk, sugar, and coconut milk in a large-sized bowl until all the ingredients are blended. Soak the bread slices in this mixture and set on the side for 2 minutes.
2. Place the grill grate inside the Ninja Foodi unit and close the hood.
3. Choose the 'GRILL' option and pick the 'MED' grill selection. Set the timer for 4 minutes and press the START/STOP button to initiate the preheating process.
4. Once the unit beeps and is ready to cook, arrange the soaked bread slice on the grill grate and cook for 2 minutes. After 2 minutes, open the grill hood to flip the bread over.
5. Proceed to cook the slices for the remainder of the cooking time.
6. Once the cooking is complete, transfer the grilled bread to separate serving plates.
7. Arrange the pineapple slices on the grill grate and repeat the above selection process. Set the timer for 4 minutes and close the lid. At the halfway mark, turn the pineapple slices over and cook for the remaining two minutes.
8. Arrange the grilled pineapple slices on the bread, sprinkle generously with coconut flakes, and serve.

GRILLED BACON SANDWICH

PREP TIME: 10 MINS | COOK TIME: 10 MINS | SERVES 4

INGREDIENTS:

- Sea salt (as required)
- Black pepper (freshly ground, as required)
- 8 tbsp. Mayonnaise
- 2 tbsp. Canola oil
- 8 Iceberg lettuce leaves
- 2 Tomatoes (sliced, with ¼ inch thickness)
- 8 Bacon slices (cooked)
- 8 Bread slices

DIRECTIONS:

1. Place the grill grate inside the Foodi grill and secure the lid. Choose the 'GRILL' option and set the timer for 10 minutes at MAX temperature. Press the START/STOP button to commence preheating.
2. Next, spread an even layer of mayonnaise on one side of each bread slice.
3. Once the unit beeps and is ready to cook, arrange the bread slices on the grill grate. Make sure to keep the mayonnaise side facing the grill grate. Secure the hood and cook for 3 minutes until the bread is ready and crisp.
4. Next, remove the seeds from the tomatoes. Brush both sides of the tomato slices with oil and sprinkle lightly with black pepper and salt.
5. Once 3 minutes have passed, take out the bread slices from the grill. Arrange the tomato slices on the grill grate and cook for 6-8 minutes.
6. To prepare the sandwich, spread an even coat of mayonnaise on the un-grilled side of the bread slices. Then proceed to layer the sandwich with lettuce, tomatoes, and bacon. Cover the sandwich with the remaining slices of bread. Cut the sandwich into equal halves and arrange on a serving plate.

HEARTY SPINACH & PORK

PREP TIME: 10 MINS | COOK TIME: 10 MINS | SERVES 2

INGREDIENTS:

- Sea salt (as required)
- 1 tbsp. Olive oil
- 1 tbsp. Canola oil (for greasing)
- 4 Eggs (medium-sized)
- 1 Red onion (sliced)
- 1 cup Button mushrooms (quartered)
- 2 cups Baby spinach
- 4 Pork sausage links

DIRECTIONS:

1. Place the grill grate inside the Foodi grill, secure the hood, and set the timer for 5 minutes at MAX temperature. Press the START/STOP button to start the preheating process.
2. Once the unit beeps and is ready to cook, arrange the sausages in the grill grate and cook for 2 minutes.
3. After 2 minutes have passed, flip the pork sausages and cook for the remainder of the time. Once the cooking cycle is over, take the sausage links out from the grill and place them on a plate. Make sure to remove the grill grate.
4. Next, grease the Ninja multi-purpose pan with canola oil. Evenly spread out the mushrooms, spinach, onions, and sausages in the pan. Crack the eggs between the pork sausages, and place the pan inside the cooking pot.
5. Select the 'BAKE' option and set the timer for 5 minutes at 350°F. Press the START/STOP button, secure the grill hood, and cook until 5 minutes are up. Serve the dish while it's warm.

CHERRY GRANOLA WITH NUTS

PREP TIME: 15 MINS | COOK TIME: 10 MINS | SERVES 4

INGREDIENTS:

- 1 tsp. Vanilla extract
- 6 tbsp. Vegetable oil
- ½ tsp. Cinnamon (ground)
- ¼ Nutmeg (ground)
- 1/3 cup Brown sugar
- ½ cup. Maple syrup (equally divided)
- 9 oz. Rolled oats
- 1 ½ cups. Almonds (untoasted, roughly chopped)
- 1 ½ cups Pistachios (salted, roughly chopped)
- 6.2 oz. Dried cherries (whole or roughly chopped)

DIRECTIONS:

1. Add the brown sugar, maple syrup, vanilla extract, cinnamon, cardamom, and vegetable oil in an adequately-sized bowl and mix until the ingredients have combined.
2. Add the oats, almonds, pistachios, and maple syrup sauce in the Ninja Grill cooking pot. Stir the mixture until the ingredients are coated in syrup.
3. Place the cooking pot inside the unit and set the timer for 20 minutes at 392°F. Secure the hood, and press the START/STOP button to commence cooking. After 12 minutes, give the granola mixture a good stir, and continue to stir at 3-minute intervals or until the granola is golden brown.
4. Once the cooking cycle is complete, place the granola on a flat pan lined with a baking sheet. Use a spatula or spoon to spread the granola across the pan's surface. Once the granola is at room temperature, sprinkle the dried cherries on top. Remember to store the granola in an air-tight container when completely cooled.

POULTRY

CHICKEN & MUSHROOM PUFF PIE

PREP TIME: 15 MINS | COOK TIME: 15 MINS | SERVES 4

INGREDIENTS:

- Salt and pepper (as required)
- 1 Egg yolk
- 2 tbsp. Olive oil (light)
- 2 tbsp. Dijon mustard
- 9.63 oz. Béchamel sauce (ready-made)
- 1 ½ tsp. Parsley (finely chopped)
- 1 ½ tsp. Tarragon (finely chopped)
- 4 Sprigs of thyme (leaves only)
- 1 leek (large, finely chopped)
- 10.5 oz. Chestnut mushrooms (halved or quartered according to size)
- 2.1 oz. Chunky smoked bacon
- 10.5 oz. Chicken thighs (boneless, roughly cut into 1/2-inch chunks)
- 7 oz. All-butter puff pastry (refrigerated)

DIRECTIONS:

1. In a large-sized bowl, add the mushrooms, thyme, leeks, chicken chunks, and bacon. Season the ingredients with oil, salt, and pepper.
2. Remove the crisper basket and grill grate from the Foodi unit. Choose the 'ROAST' option and set the timer for 15 minutes at 374°F. Press the START/STOP button to let the unit preheat.
3. When you hear the unit beep, transfer the content of the bowl to the cooking pot, and stir to spread out the ingredients. Secure the hood and allow the cooking cycle to begin.
4. After 8 minutes, open the grill hood and stir the contents. At the 12 minute mark, check to see if the ingredients are cooked. If additional cooking is required, stir the contents and secure the hood to cook for the remainder of the time.
5. Remove the chicken from the cooking pot after it's cooked, and transfer it to a bowl with the sauce. Wash the cooking pot, dry it, and place it back in the Foodi unit.
6. Add mustard, herbs, and béchamel sauce to the chicken. Taste the mixture to see if additional seasoning is required. Set the bowl aside to allow the mixture to cool.
7. Once you're ready to bake, use a 7-inch pie tin (or a 3-inch deep-dish) to transfer the filling.
8. On a clean work surface, roll out the pastry to a 9-inch circle with 0.19-inch thickness. Refrigerate the pastry for 15 minutes. Combine 1 ½ tsp. of water, a pinch of salt, and the egg yolk to create the egg wash.
9. Brush the edge or lip of the pastry dish with the egg wash to allow the pastry to stick to it. Carefully place the rolled out pastry circle on top of the filling and lightly press the edges with a fork to make indents. Brush the top of the pastry with the egg wash. Remember to prick a few holes in the pastry, with the fork.
10. Choose the 'BAKE' option and set the timer for 25 minutes at 374°F. Press the START/STOP button to allow the unit to preheat.
11. Once you hear the unit beep, open the grill hood, and carefully place the pie dish into the cooking pot. Secure the hood and allow the pastry to cook. At the 10-minutes mark, reduce the temperature to 338°F, and continue cooking.
12. When the cooking cycle is complete, carefully lift the pie out of the unit with the help of oven gloves or mitts. Serve the pie while it's hot.

STICKY HONEY CHICKEN THIGHS

PREP TIME: 5 MINS | COOK TIME: 15 MINS | SERVES 4

INGREDIENTS:

- Juice of 2 limes
- 1 cup Sriracha sauce
- ¼ cup Honey
- 4 Chicken thighs (with bone)

DIRECTIONS:

1. Add the honey, sriracha sauce, and lemon juice in a large-sized resealable bag. Next, add the chicken thighs, seal the bag, and gently shake it to coat the chicken in the sticky honey sauce. Place the bag in the refrigerator for 30 minutes.
2. Place the grill grate inside the Foodi grill. Choose the 'GRILL' option and set the timer for 14 minutes at MEDIUM temperature. Press the START/STOP button to initiate the preheating process.
3. When the unit is ready to cook and emits a beeping sound, open the grill hood and arrange the chicken thighs on the grill grate. Gently press down on the chicken meat to ensure grill marks. Secure the hood and cook for 7 minutes.
4. Turn the chicken thighs after 7 minutes using tongs. Close the grill lid and cook for the remainder of the time.
5. When the timer runs out, transfer the chicken thighs to a cutting board and allow to rest for 5 minutes. After that serve the sticky honey thighs immediately.

CREAMY CHICKEN ZUCCHINI KEBABS

PREP TIME: 15 MINS | COOK TIME: 15 MINS | SERVES 4

INGREDIENTS:

- 1 tsp. Sea salt
- ½ tsp. Black pepper (freshly ground)
- ¼ cup Greek yogurt (plain)
- ¼ cup Olive oil (extra virgin)
- Juice of 4 lemons
- Zest of 1 lemon
- 4 Garlic cloves (finely chopped)
- 2 tbsp. Thyme (dried)
- 1 Onion (quartered)
- 1 Zucchini (sliced)
- 1 lb. Skinless chicken breasts (cut into 2-inch cubes)

DIRECTIONS:

1. Whisk the lemon juice, olive oil, Greek yogurt, salt, pepper, thyme, garlic, and lemon zest in a large-sized bowl, until the ingredients are mixed well.
2. Add the chicken cubes and half the yogurt marinade in a large resealable bag. Gently shake the sealed back to coat the chicken in the marinade. Place in the refrigerator for 30 minutes.
3. Place the grill grate inside the Foodi grill. Choose the 'GRILL' option and set the timer for 14 minutes at MEDIUM temperature. Press the START/START button to allow the unit to preheat.
4. Next, make the kebabs by attaching the chicken cubes to the skewers. Make sure to switch the chicken with zucchini and onion while threading. Remember to push the ingredients towards the end of the skewers.
5. Once the unit beeps, arrange the skewers on the grill grate and close the hood. Cook for 10 to 14 minutes and baste the kebabs with the yogurt marinade once every three to four minutes while cooking.
6. Once the internal temperature of the kebabs reads 165°F on the food thermometer, it's ready to serve.

CHEESE & CHICKEN QUESADILLA

PREP TIME: 10 MINS | COOK TIME: 40 MINS | SERVES 4

INGREDIENTS:

- Cooking spray
- 5 drops Hot sauce
- 5 1/8 tbsp. Sour cream
- 5 1/8 tbsp. Salsa
- 3.5 oz. can of diced jalapeño peppers
- 5 Spring onions (chopped, divided as per directions)
- 19 oz. Cheddar (grated, divided as per directions)
- 4 Flour tortillas

DIRECTIONS:

1. Place the grill grate inside the unit and secure the lid. Choose the 'GRILL' option and set the timer for 4 minutes at MAX temperature. Press the START/STOP button to allow the unit to preheat.
2. Spray both sides of the tortillas with cooking spray and poke 5 to 6 holes in them with a knife tip.
3. Mix the salsa, sour cream, and hot sauce in a small-sized bowl, and set aside.
4. When you hear the unit beep, place 1 tortilla on the grill grate and cook for 1 minute. Remove the tortilla from the grate and set aside. Repeat this process for the remaining tortillas.
5. Place a tortilla on a flat work surface, and top with 1/3 of the chicken, spring onions, jalapeño peppers, and salsa mixture. Add 5.6 oz. of grated cheese. Next, place another tortilla on top of the filling. Repeat the filling and topping process (with the same quantity of ingredients) twice more. In the end, you should have a stack of 4 tortillas.
6. Take the grill grate out of the unit. Choose the 'ROAST' option and set the timer for 23 minutes at 356°F. Press the START/STOP button to allow the grill unit to preheat.
7. When you hear the unit beep, carefully place the tortilla stack in the cooking pot and cover it with aluminum foil, and secure the sides. Close the grill hood and cook for 20 minutes. Sprinkle the remaining cheese on top of the quesadilla stack and cook for an additional 3 minutes.
8. Once the cooking cycle is complete, remove the quesadilla stack from the grill, and transfer to a serving plate. Slice and serve.

TERIYAKI CHICKEN KEBABS

PREP TIME: 15 MINS | COOK TIME: 15 MINS | SERVES 4

INGREDIENTS:

- 1 cup Teriyaki sauce (divided as per directions)
- 2 cups Fresh pineapple (cut into 1-inch cubes)
- 2 Green bell pepper (de-seeded, cut to 1-inch cubes)
- 1 lb. Skinless chicken breasts (cut into 2-inch cubes)

DIRECTIONS:

1. Add the teriyaki sauce and chicken in an adequately-sized container. Cover the lid and gently shake the container to coat the chicken in sauce. Place in the refrigerator for 30 minutes.
2. Place the grill grate inside the Foodi grill and secure the hood. Choose the 'GRILL' option and set the timer for 14 minutes at MEDIUM temperature. Press the START/STOP button to allow the unit to preheat.
3. Next, start assembling the kebabs by threading chicken, pepper, and pineapple cubes alternatively. Make sure to push the ingredients towards the end of the skewer.
4. Once the unit beeps, put the skewers on the grill grate and secure the hood. Cook the kebabs for 14 minutes, and baste them every 4 minutes with the teriyaki marinade.
5. Once the cooking cycle is complete, the internal temperature of the kebabs should read 165°F on a food thermometer.

SPICY CHICKEN KEBABS

PREP TIME: 15 MINS | COOK TIME: 15 MINS | SERVES 4

INGREDIENTS:

- ¼ tsp. Sea salt
- 2 tsp. Paprika
- 1 tbsp. Garlic powder
- 1 tbsp. Cumin (ground)
- 1 tbsp. Chili powder
- 2 tbsp. Olive oil (extra-virgin, divided as per directions)
- 1 Onion (quartered)
- 2 Red bell peppers (de-seeded, cut into 1-inch cubes)
- Juice of 1 lime
- 1 lb. Skinless chicken breasts (cut into 2-inch cubes)

DIRECTIONS:

1. Add garlic powder, salt, chili powder, cumin, and paprika in a small-sized bowl. Mix the ingredients with a spoon.
2. Next, put 1 tbsp. of oil, half of the spice mixture, and chicken cubes in a large resealable bag. Gently shake the bag after sealing to coat the chicken in spices.
3. Place the onions and bell peppers in another resealable bag with 1 tbsp. of oil and the remaining spice mixture. Shake the bag gently after sealing it to coat the vegetables in spices. Place the spiced vegetables and chicken in the refrigerator for 30 minutes.
4. Place the grill grate inside the Foodi grill and choose the 'GRILL' option. Set the timer for 14 minutes and set the temperature to HIGH. Press the START/STOP button to start the preheating process.
5. Next, assemble the kebabs by threading the chicken cubes, pepper, and onions alternatively on the skewers. Make sure to push the ingredients towards the end of the skewers.
6. Once the unit beeps, arrange the skewers on the grill grate and cook for 14 minutes.
7. Once the cooking cycle is complete, the internal temperature of the chicken kebabs should be no less than 165°F. If the temperature is lower, continue to cook the kebabs for an additional minute. Once the kebabs are ready, drizzle them with lemon juice, and enjoy!

CRISPY WINGS

PREP TIME: 5 MINS | COOK TIME: 25 MINS | SERVES 4

INGREDIENTS:

- Sea salt (as required)
- Black pepper (freshly ground, as required)
- 1 ½ tbsp. Cooking oil
- 1 ½ cup Dill pickle juice
- ½ tbsp. dried dill
- ¾ tsp. Garlic (minced)
- 2 lbs. Chicken wings

DIRECTIONS:

1. In a large-sized bowl, soaked the chicken wings in dill pickle juice. Make sure to coat the meat thoroughly. Cover the bowl and place in the refrigerator for 2 hours.
2. Place the crisper basket in the Ninja Foodi Grill, and secure the hood. Choose the 'AIR CRISP' option and set the timer for 26 minutes at 390°F. Press the START/STOP button to initiate the preheating process.
3. Next, take the chicken wings out of the dill juice, and rinse them with cold water. Place the wings in another bowl after patting them dry with a paper towel.
4. Whisk the dried dill, oil, garlic, salt, and pepper in a small-sized bowl. Once the ingredients have combined, drizzle the mixture over the chicken wings. Toss the chicken wings in the mixture to ensure an even coat.
5. Once the preheating cycle is complete and the unit beeps, arrange the wings in the crisper basket. Make sure not to place the wings too close to each other. Secure the grill hood and cook for 11 minutes.
6. Once 11 minutes are up, open the hood and turn the wings with the help of tongs. Secure the hood and allow the wings to cook for another 11 minutes.
7. Once the timer runs out, check to see if the wings are done. The internal temperature of the meat should read 165°F (at least) on the food thermometer for the chicken wings to be ready. If necessary, cook the wings for an additional 4 minutes.
8. Once the wings are ready, transfer to a serving plate and serve.

ROSEMARY GRILLED CHICKEN

PREP TIME: 10 MINS | COOK TIME: 15 MINS | SERVES 4

INGREDIENTS:

- Sea salt (as required)
- 1/8 tsp. black pepper
- Juice of 2 lemons (freshly squeezed)
- Zest of 2 lemons
- ¼ cup Olive oil
- 2 Garlic cloves (finely chopped)
- ¼ tsp. Red pepper flakes
- 3 Sprigs of sage (leaves only, minced)
- 3 sprlgs rosemary (leaves only, minced)
- 4-7 oz. Boneless chicken thighs

DIRECTIONS:

1. Whisk the lemon juice, sage, rosemary, lemon zest, red pepper flakes, garlic, pepper and oil in a small-size bowl. Season the marinade with salt.
2. Add the marinade and chicken thighs in a resealable bag. Seal the bag and shake it gently to coat the chicken in the marinade. Place in the refrigerator for 30 minutes.
3. Put the grill grate inside the Foodi Grill and secure the hood. Choose the 'GRILL' option and set the timer for 13 minutes at HIGH temperature. Press the START/STOP button to allow the unit to preheat.
4. Once the unit beeps and is ready to cook, arrange the chicken thighs on the grill grate, and close the lid. Cook the chicken for 13 minutes.
5. Once the cooking cycle is finished, check the chicken for doneness. The internal temperature of the chicken thighs should read 165°F on the food thermometer for the chicken to be done.

JALAPENO BURGER

PREP TIME: 5 MINS | COOK TIME: 15 MINS | SERVES 4

INGREDIENTS:

- ½ tsp. Sea salt
- ½ tsp. Black pepper (freshly ground)
- 1 tsp. Paprika
- 1 ½ tsp. Cumin (ground)
- 3 tbsp. Bread crumbs
- 1 Jalapeño pepper (de-seeded, finely chopped)

- ½ Onion (finely chopped)
- 4 Burger buns
- 1 lb. Turkey (ground)
- Cheese, lettuce, tomatoes (for serving)
- Mustard, ketchup (for serving)

DIRECTIONS:

1. Place the grill grate inside the Foodi Grill and secure the hood. Choose the 'GRILL' option and set the timer for 13 minutes at HIGH temperature. Press the START/STOP button to allow the unit to preheat.
2. In a large-sized bowl, add the ground turkey, bread crumbs, jalapeño pepper, onion, cumin, paprika, salt, and pepper. Use your hand to combine the ingredients. However, do not overwork the mixture.
3. To make the turkey burger patties, lightly wet your hands with cold water, and form 4 burger patties of equal size.
4. Once the unit beeps and is ready to cook, arrange the burgers on the grill grate, and secure the hood. Cook the patties for 11 minutes.
5. Once 11 minutes have passed, check the internal temperature of the patties. If the reading on the food thermometer is lower than 165°F, then cook for another 2 minutes.
6. Once the patties are well cooked, transfer them to the burger buns and proceed to prepare your burger to your preference with lettuce, cheese, and tomatoes. Serve with ketchup or mustard.

LIME & BLACK PEPPER CHICKEN

PREP TIME: 5 MINS | COOK TIME: 20 MINS | SERVES 4

INGREDIENTS:

- Sea salt (as required)
- Black pepper (freshly ground, as required)
- 1 ½ tbsp. Olive oil (extra virgin)
- Juice of 1 lime
- Zest of 1 lime
- 3 Garlic cloves (minced)

- 4 Boneless chicken breasts
- Zest of 1 lime
- 3 Garlic cloves (minced)
- 4 Boneless chicken breasts

DIRECTIONS:

1. Whisk the garlic, salt, pepper, lemon juice, zest, and oil in a large-sized bowl. Add the chicken breasts and turn them to coat the meat with the marinade. Cover and place the bowl in the refrigerator for 30 minutes.
2. Place the grill grate inside the Ninja Foodi Grill and choose the 'GRILL' option. Set the timer for 18 minutes at MEDIUM temperature. Press the START/STOP button to allow the unit to preheat.
3. Once the unit beeps, arrange the chicken breasts on the grate, and allow them to cook for 7 minutes. Once 7 minutes are up, open the grill hood, turn the chicken breasts, and cook for an additional 7 minutes.
4. After 7 minutes, check to see if the chicken is done. If more cooking is required, cook for 4 more minutes. The chicken will be ready when the internal temperature reads a minimum of 165°F on a food thermometer.
5. Next, transfer the chicken breasts to a cutting board to rest for at least 5 minutes. Serve while still warm.

TERIYAKI WINGS

PREP TIME: 5 MINS | COOK TIME: 15 MINS | SERVES 4

INGREDIENTS:

- 1 cup Honey
- 1/4 cup Teriyaki sauce
- 1/3 cup Soy sauce
- 2 tsp. Garlic powder
- 1 tsp. Black pepper (freshly ground)
- 3 Garlic cloves (finely chopped)
- 2 lbs. Chicken wings

DIRECTIONS:

1. Place the grill grate inside the Foodi Grill and secure the hood. Choose the 'GRILL' option and set the timer for 14 minutes at MEDIUM temperature. Press the START/STOP button to start the preheating process.
2. Whisk the honey, teriyaki sauce, soy sauce, garlic powder, garlic, and black pepper in a large bowl. Next, add chicken wings to the bowl and use tongs to coat the wings in the sauce thoroughly.
3. When the unit beeps and is ready to cook, arrange the chicken wings on the grill grate. Secure the hood and cook for minutes. When 5 minutes are up, open the hood to turn the chicken wings and cook for another 5 minutes.
4. Check if the wings are done once the cooking cycle is over. To be perfectly cooked, the internal temperature of the meat must be 165°F (at least) on a food thermometer. If the reading is lower, then cook the wings for an additional 4 minutes.
5. After 4 minutes have passed, transfer the wings to a serving plate, and enjoy.

CRUMBLED BUTTERED CHICKEN

PREP TIME: 5 MINS | COOK TIME: 25 MINS | SERVES 2

INGREDIENTS:

- 2 Eggs (large)
- ½ tsp. Black pepper (freshly ground)
- Juice of 1 lemon
- 1 tbsp. Green olives (sliced, drained)
- 4 tbsp. Butter (unsalted)
- ½ cup All-purpose flour
- 2 Chicken breasts (boneless, skinless)

DIRECTIONS:

1. Place the crisper basket inside the grill unit and secure the hood. Choose the 'AIR CRISP' option and set the timer for 22 minutes at 375°F. Press the START/STOP button to allow the unit to preheat.
2. Whisk the eggs in a medium-sized bowl until they are beaten well.
3. In another medium-sized bowl, add the black pepper and flour and mix together using a fork.
4. Next, add the chicken to the flour and coat it properly. Then dip the chicken breasts in the egg, and return to the flour.
5. Once the unit beeps and is ready to cook, arrange the chicken breasts in the crisper basket and secure the hood to cook for 18 minutes.
6. Proceed to melt butter in a skillet over a medium flame, and add the green olives and lemon juice once the butter turns light brown. Reduce the heat, and let the butter sauce cook for 3 to 4 minutes. Remove from heat once done.
7. Check to see if the chicken breasts are ready once 18 minutes are up. The internal temperature of the chicken needs to be 165°F on a food thermometer. If the reading is lower than that, then cook the chicken for an additional 3 minutes.
8. Once the cooking cycle is over, transfer the chicken to a serving plate and drizzle with the butter and green olive sauce to serve.

RED PEPPER ROASTED CHICKEN

PREP TIME: 10 MINS | COOK TIME: 25 MINS | SERVES 4

INGREDIENTS:

- 1/3 cup Olive oil
- ½ tsp. Salt
- 2 tsp. Cumin (ground)
- 2 tsp. Paprika
- 1/2 cup Flat-leaf parsley (finely chopped)
- 3 Garlic cloves (finely chopped, equally divided)
- 3 tbsp. Yogurt (plain)
- 4 Chicken thighs (skinless & boneless)

DIRECTIONS:

1. Add the yogurt, garlic, oil, and salt to a blender and blend until a smooth mixture forms. Place the mixture inside the refrigerator.
2. In a large-sized bowl, add the paprika, parsley, garlic, and cumin. Mix the ingredients well and add the chicken thighs. Make sure the meat is well coated with the spices. Place the bowl inside the refrigerator for 2 to 4 hours.
3. Place the cooking pot inside the Ninja Foodi Grill, and grease its surface with cooking spray.
4. Choose the 'ROAST' option and set the timer for 23 minutes at 400°F. Press the START/STOP button to allow the unit to preheat.
5. Once the unit beeps and is ready to cook, open the grill hood and add the chicken thighs to the cooking pot. Secure the hood and cook for 15 minutes.
6. After 15 minutes, open the grill hood, and turn the chicken over. Secure the top and cook for an additional 8 minutes.
7. Transfer the chicken to serving plates once the cooking cycle is over and serve with the yogurt sauce.

TANGY BBQ DRUMSTICKS

PREP TIME: 5 MINS | COOK TIME: 20 MINS | SERVES 4

INGREDIENTS:

- Sea salt (as required)
- Black pepper (as required)
- 2 cup Barbecue sauce
- Juice of 1 lemon
- 1 tbsp. Tabasco
- 1 lb. Chicken drumsticks

DIRECTIONS:

1. In a large-sized bowl, mix the lemon juice, honey, barbecue sauce, salt, and pepper. Whisk the ingredients until well combined. Take out ½ of the sauce mixture and set aside. Next, add the chicken drumsticks to the bowl and toss gently to make sure the drumsticks are coated.
2. Place the grill grate inside the Foodi grill and choose the 'GRILL' options. Set the timer for 20 minutes at MEDIUM temperature. Press the START/STOP button to allow the unit to preheat.
3. Once the unit beeps and is ready to cook, arrange the drumsticks on the grill grate, secure the hood, and cook for 18 minutes. Make sure to baste the drumsticks at regular intervals during this time.
4. The drumsticks will be ready when the internal temperature of the meat reads 165°F (at least) on a food thermometer. If required, cook the chicken drumsticks for another 2 minutes to ensure doneness.

PAPRIKA CHICKEN CUTLETS

PREP TIME: 5 MINS | COOK TIME: 11 MINS | SERVES 2

INGREDIENTS:

- ½ tbsp. Olive oil (extra virgin)
- ¼ tsp. Sea salt
- ¼ tsp. Garlic powder
- ¼ tsp. Paprika
- ¼ tsp. Black pepper (freshly ground)
- 1/8 cup Bread crumbs
- 1/2 lb. Chicken breasts (boneless & skinless, sliced crosswise in half)

DIRECTIONS:

1. Place the crisper basket in the Foodi Grill and secure the hood. Choose the 'AIR CRISP' option and set the timer for 11 minutes at 375°F. Press the START/STOP button to allow the unit to preheat.
2. Brush the cutlets (overall) with oil.
3. In a large-sized bowl, combine the bread crumbs, paprika, salt, pepper, and garlic powder. Add the chicken cutlets to the bread crumbs and turn over several times to make sure the chicken is coated evenly on all sides.
4. When you heat the unit beep, arrange the chicken cutlets in the crisper basket. Secure the grill hood and cook for 9 minutes. The chicken will be ready when the internal temperature reads 165°F (at least) on a food thermometer. If the reading is lower, then cook the cutlets for an additional 2 minutes.
5. When the cooking cycle is done, transfer the cutlets to a serving plate and serve.

BBQ BEER WINGS

PREP TIME: 15 MINS | COOK TIME: 35 MINS | SERVES 2

INGREDIENTS:

- Sea salt (as required)
- Black pepper (freshly ground, as required)
- 2 tbsp. Canola oil
- ½ cup Barbecue sauce
- 1 tbsp. Garlic powder
- 1 tsp. Onion powder
- ½ cup Beer
- 1 lb. Chicken wings

DIRECTIONS:

1. In a large-sized bowl, combine all the ingredients (except wings) and mix well. Once the mixture is ready, add the chicken wings and coat them well on all sides.
2. Place the grill grate inside the Foodi Grill and secure the lid. Choose the 'GRILL' option and set the time for 25 minutes at MEDIUM temperature. Press the START/STOP button to allow the unit to preheat.
3. Once the unit beeps and is ready to cook, arrange the chicken wings on the grill grate and set the marinade aside. Secure the grill hood and cook for 13 minutes.
4. After 13 minutes are up, open the hood and turn the chicken wings over. Cook for another 12 minutes.
5. When 12 minutes have passed, open the grill hood and carefully take the grill grate out with the help of oven gloves/mitts.
6. Place the cooking pot inside the grill unit and add the marinade sauce. Secure the grill and choose the 'ROAST' option. Set the timer for 15 minutes at 350°F. Press the START/STOP button to commence cooking.
7. Cook the marinade sauce for 15 minutes. Then transfer the chicken wings to a serving plate and serve with the sauce.

ORANGE TURMERIC CHICKEN

PREP TIME: 10 MINS | COOK TIME: 25 MINS | SERVES 4

INGREDIENTS:

- 4 tbsp. Olive oil (extra virgin)
- 4 oz. Orange juice
- 1 tbsp. Vinegar
- 2 tsp. turmeric powder
- 2 tsp. Oregano
- ½ tsp. Black pepper (freshly ground)
- 4 Garlic cloves (finely chopped)
- 4 Chicken breasts (boneless)

DIRECTIONS:

1. In a large-sized bowl, combine all the ingredients (except chicken) and mix well. Next, add the chicken and coat well on all sides. Cover the bowl and refrigerate it for 2 to 3 hours.
2. Place the grill grate inside the Foodi Grill, and secure the hood. Choose the 'GRILL' option and set the timer for 22 minutes at MEDIUM temperature. Press the START/STOP button to allow the unit to preheat.
3. Once the unit beeps and is ready to cook, open the grill hood, and arrange the chicken on the grill grate.
4. Secure the hood yet again, and cook for 11 minutes. After 11 minutes have passed, turn the chicken over and cook for the remainder of the time.
5. Once the cooking cycle is finished, transfer the chicken to a serving plate and serve warm.

GRILLED CHICKEN WITH PEANUT SAUCE

PREP TIME: 15 MINS | COOK TIME: 10 MINS | SERVES 4

INGREDIENTS:

- Cooking Spray
- ½ tsp. Salt
- 2 tsp. Brown sugar
- 1 tbsp. Canola oil
- 1 tbsp. Water
- 1 ½ tbsp. Rice vinegar
- ½ tsp. Chili powder
- 2 tsp. Sriracha sauce
- ½ tsp. Garlic powder
- 1 tsp. Ginger (finely chopped)
- 1 Garlic clove (finely chopped)
- ¼ cup Cilantro leaves
- ¼ cup Peanut Butter (creamy)
- 4 Chicken breast halves (skinless & boneless, 6 oz. each)

DIRECTIONS:

1. In a large-sized bowl, add the salt, brown sugar, and chili powder and mix well. Next, add the chicken breasts to the spice mixture and coat evenly on all sides.
2. Place the grill grate inside the Ninja Foodi Grill, and secure the hood. Choose the 'GRILL' option and set the timer for 5 minutes on HIGH temperature. Press the START/STOP button to allow the grill to preheat.
3. Once the unit beeps, open the hood and grease the grill grate with cooking spray. Arrange the chicken on the grill grate and cook for 5 minutes. At the halfway mark, open the hood to turn the chicken breasts over. Once done, secure the hood and cook for the remainder of the time.
4. Once the cooking time is complete, transfer the chicken to a cutting board and allow it to rest for 5 minutes. Next, proceed to slice the chicken breasts.
5. In an adequately-sized bowl, add the peanut butter, chili powder, oil, water, rice vinegar, sriracha sauce, ginger, garlic, and cilantro leaves. Use a whisk to blend the ingredients. Drizzle the peanut sauce generously over the chicken slices when you serve and garnish with cilantro leaves.

BOURBON CHICKEN

PREP TIME: 10 MINS | COOK TIME: 15 MINS | SERVES 4

INGREDIENTS:

- Salt (as required)
- 1 tbsp. Brown sugar
- 1 tbsp. Bourbon
- 2 tsp. Barbecue seasoning
- 1/2 cup Ketchup
- 1/3 cup mixed spice
- 1 tsp. Dried onion (minced)
- 6 Chicken drumsticks

DIRECTIONS:

1. Add all the ingredients (except drumsticks) to an adequately-sized saucepan, and cook for 8 to 10 minutes. Set the pan aside for the sauce to cool.
2. Place the grill grate inside the Foodi Grill and secure the hood. Choose the 'GRILL' option and set the timer for 12 minutes at MEDIUM temperature. Press the START/STOP button to allow the unit to preheat.
3. Once the unit beeps and the preheating process is completed, open the grill hood and arrange the drumsticks over the grill grate. Next, brush the drumsticks with the sauce, secure the lid and cook for 6 minutes.
4. After 6 minutes are over, open the hood and turn the drumsticks. Brush the drumsticks with the remaining sauce, and cook for another 6 minutes.
5. Once the cooking cycle is done, the drumsticks are ready to serve.

HOT & SPICY CHICKEN

PREP TIME: 60 MINS | COOK TIME: 30 MINS | SERVES 4

INGREDIENTS:

For the chicken
- Salt (as required)
- Juice of ½ a lemon
- 3 Garlic cloves (crushed)
- 4 Whole chicken legs (with skin)

Hot & Spicy Sauce
- 1.7 oz. Olive oil
- 1.7 oz. Lemon juice
- 2 Garlic cloves (minced)
- ¼ tsp. Chili powder
- ½ tsp. Cayenne powder

For garlic bread
- Salt (as required)
- 2 Garlic cloves (finely chopped)
- Olive oil (as required)
- 2 tsp. Oregano
- 2 French baguettes

DIRECTIONS:

1. Prepare the marinade by mixing lemon juice, salt, and garlic in a large-sized bowl. Add the chicken and coat it well in the marinade. Cover the bowl and place it in the refrigerator for 1 hour.
2. Place the grill grate inside the Foodi grill and secure the hood. Choose the 'GRILL' option and set the timer for 30 minutes at HIGH temperature. Press the START/STOP button to start the preheating process.
3. Once the unit beeps and is ready to cook, arrange the chicken on the grill grate (skin side down) and sprinkle with salt. Secure the hood and cook for 10 minutes.
4. After 10 minutes have passed; check to see how the chicken is doing. The skin should look nicely browned. Turn the chicken over and cook for 10 more minutes. While the chicken is cooking, combine all the ingredients for the hot and spicy sauce in a bowl and whisk well.
5. Open the grill hood, brush the top side of the chicken legs with the hot and spicy sauce and then turn the pieces over. Cook the chicken for 5 minutes, and keep brushing the meat with the sauce at regular intervals.
6. After 5 minutes, check if the meat is cooked through, by using the tip of a knife to prick the chicken leg near the joint. Transfer the chicken legs to a warmed plate.
7. Proceed to secure the grill hood and set the timer for 6 minutes at MEDIUM temperature. In a small-sized bowl, mix the ingredients listed for the garlic bread and whisk until well combined. Make 5 or 6 crosswise cuts on the baguette, and use a brush to generously spread the garlic sauce inside the bread between the cuts. Place the bread on the grill grate and cook for 3 to 5 minutes or until the bread is lightly browned.

EASY STUFFED CHICKEN WITH VEGGIES

PREP TIME: 5 MINS | COOK TIME: 45 MINS | SERVES 4

INGREDIENTS:

- Salt (as required)
- Black pepper (freshly ground, as required)
- 1 tbsp. Olive oil (extra virgin)
- 1 tsp. Oregano
- 0.7 oz. Parmesan (shredded)
- 1 tbsp. Fresh parsley (finely chopped)
- 1 Courgette (roughly chopped)
- 1 Red bell pepper (de-seeded, sliced with 1/4-inch thickness)
- 1 Yellow bell pepper (de-seeded, sliced with 1/4-inch thickness)
- 1 Garlic clove (diced)
- 4 Ham slices
- 4 Chicken breasts

DIRECTIONS:

1. Begin with trimming the chicken breasts, then butterfly them and slightly flatten with a mallet. Sprinkle black pepper and salt on both sides.
2. Spatter parmesan generously on one side of the chicken breast, and 1 slice of ham on the other. Sprinkle the finely chopped parsley on top and carefully roll the chicken. Secure the chicken by adding toothpicks at the ends.
3. Place the grill grate inside the grill unit. Choose the 'GRILL' option and set the timer for 25 minutes at MEDIUM temperature. Press the START/STOP button to allow the unit to preheat.
4. Next, in a large-sized bowl, add the bell peppers, courgette, garlic, salt, pepper, and olive oil. Toss to ensure all the vegetables are well coated and seasoned.
5. When the unit beeps and is ready to cook, arrange the rolls on the grill grate carefully and secure the hood to cook.
6. With 10 minutes left on the timer, open the grill hood, and add the vegetables to the grate. Secure the lid, and cook for the remainder of the time.
7. When the cooking cycle is complete, transfer the rolls to a plate or board and allow them to rest for 1 to 2 minutes. Serve the rolls warm with the grilled vegetables.

FETA CHICKEN & COUSCOUS

PREP TIME: 10 MINS | COOK TIME: 25 MINS | SERVES 2

INGREDIENTS:

- Salt (as required)
- Black pepper (as required)
- 1 tbsp. Canola oil
- 2 tbsp. Tomato puree
- 1 tsp. Garlic powder
- 1 tbsp. Sriracha sauce
- 2 Tomatoes (roughly chopped)
- 1 Onion (roughly chopped)
- 1 Bell pepper (seeded, minced)
- ½ Vegetable stock cube
- 4.2 oz. Water
- 4.2 oz. Couscous
- 2 Chicken breasts (sliced)
- Feta cheese and fresh parsley for garnish

DIRECTIONS:

1. Start with boiling 4 oz. water. Add the vegetable stock cube to the water and stir until the cube dissolves. In a large-sized bowl, add the couscous and the vegetable stock. Cover the bowl and set aside.
2. Place the cooking pot inside the Foodi grill and choose the 'ROAST' option. Set the timer for 15 minutes at 392°F. Press the START/STOP button to allow the unit to preheat.
3. In a medium-sized bowl add the oil, garlic powder, salt, pepper, and oil. Mix well until the spices are combined. Add the chicken breast slices and coat well with the mixture.
4. Once the unit beeps and is ready to cook, add the chicken to the cooking pot and secure the hood to cook.
5. Add the bell pepper, onion, and tomatoes, to the cooking pot with 10 minutes left on the timer. Close the hood and continue cooking.
6. Next, add the sriracha sauce, tomato puree, couscous to the cooking pot after two minutes, and stir to combine the ingredients.
7. Once the unit is done cooking, add the parsley and stir. Transfer the chicken and couscous to a serving plate, garnish with feta and serve.

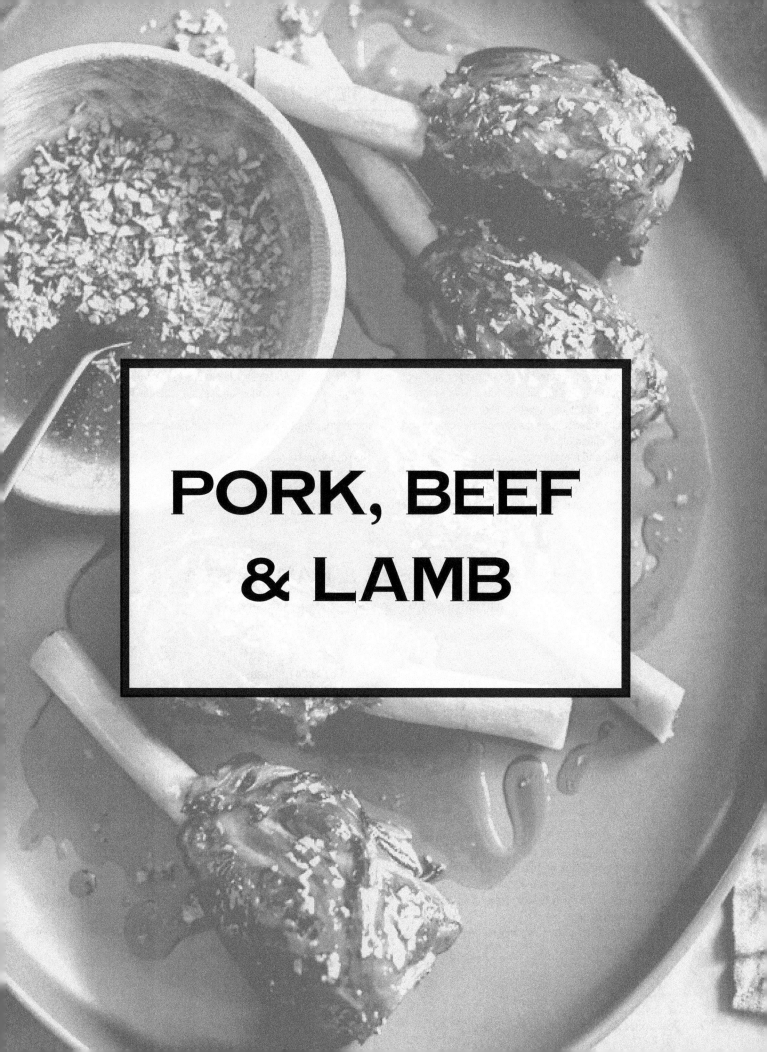

PORK, BEEF & LAMB

LOADED PORK TENDERLOIN

PREP TIME: 5 MINS | COOK TIME: 35 MINS | SERVES 4

INGREDIENTS:

- Salt (as required)
- Pepper (as required)
- 1 tbsp. Butter
- 1 tbsp. Honey
- 1 tbsp. Mayonnaise

- 1 Apple (grated)
- 10 Sage leaves (finely chopped)
- 3.5 oz. Bacon
- 1 Pork tenderloin

DIRECTIONS:

1. Start preparing your pork tenderloin by placing it on a clean cutting board and cutting a 1-inch opening through its length.
2. Combine the mayo and honey in a small bowl and mix well. Brush this mixture on the tenderloin, and make sure to brush inside the opening as well.
3. In a large-sized bowl, add the sage, butter, salt, pepper, and apple and mix with a spoon. Add the apple mixture to the pork opening.
4. Place the crisper basket inside the Ninja Foodi Grill and secure the hood. Choose the 'ROAST' option, and set the timer for 30 minutes at 464°F. Press the START/STOP button to allow the unit to preheat.
5. Next, wrap the pork tenderloin with the bacon rashers. Make sure to wrap the strips tightly around the pork and attach skewers at the ends to keep the strips from falling off.
6. When the unit beeps and is ready to cook, place the pork tenderloin on the crisper basket carefully. Secure the hood and cook for 30 minutes.
7. Brush the tenderloin with the honey and mayonnaise glaze every 10 minutes.
8. When the cooking cycle is complete, transfer the tenderloin from the grill to a cutting board and let it rest for 3 to 5 minutes.
9. Serve a succulent slice of pork tenderloin with a side of veggies and mashed potatoes.

HEARTY CHEESE & HAM PASTA

PREP TIME: 30 MINS | COOK TIME: 30 MINS | SERVES 4

INGREDIENTS:

- 4 Eggs
- 1 tsp. Salt
- 1 ½ tbsp. Butter (melted)
- ½ tsp. Nutmeg
- 1 tbsp. Fresh parsley (minced)
- 5 oz. Milk

- 7 oz. Ham (minced)
- 10 oz. Fine ribbon pasta (pre-cooked)

DIRECTIONS:

1. Place the cooking pot inside the Ninja Foodi Grill and choose the 'BAKE' option. Set the timer for 17 minutes at 356°F. Press the START/STOP button to commence the preheating process.
2. Add the ham, butter, cooked pasta, parsley, and butter in a large-sized bowl. Toss well to evenly combine the ingredients.
3. In a medium-sized bowl, add eggs, milk, salt, and nutmeg. Whisk the ingredient until combined.
4. Once the unit beeps and is ready to cook, grease the cooking pot with cooking spray. Next, add the pasta and egg mixture and stir. Secure the grill hood to commence cooking.
5. When the cooking cycle is finished, carefully remove the cooking pot with oven gloves/mitts and allow it to cool down a little. Transfer the casserole to a serving plate and serve.

SEARED STEAK SALAD WITH A CRUNCH

PREP TIME: 5 MINS | COOK TIME: 15 MINS | SERVES 5

INGREDIENTS:

- Salt (as required)
- Black pepper (freshly ground, as required)
- 1 cup Croutons
- 1 cup Blue cheese dressing
- 6 cups Romaine lettuce (chopped)
- ¾ cups Cherry tomatoes (halved)
- 2 Avocados (peeled, sliced)
- 4 Skirt steaks (8 oz. each)

DIRECTIONS:

1. Place the grill grate inside the Foodi Grill and secure the hood. Choose the 'GRILL' option and set the timer for 8 minutes at HIGH temperature. Press the START/STOP button to allow the unit to preheat.
2. Season the skirt steaks with salt and pepper on both sides.
3. When the unit beeps and is ready to cook, arrange 2 steaks on the grill grate and press down lightly to ensure grill marks. Secure the grill hood and cook for 4 minutes. After 4 minutes, open the lid and turn the steaks over. Cook for another 4 minutes.
4. Transfer the steaks to a cutting board and lightly cover with aluminum foil to keep warm.
5. Repeat the cooking process for the remaining 2 steaks.
6. Next, prepare the salad by tossing the tomatoes, lettuce, croutons in a large-sized bowl. Add the avocado slices on the top.
7. When the remaining steaks are cooked, transfer them to the cutting board and allow them to rest for a few minutes. Cut all 4 steaks into strips. Place some salad on a serving plate and top the salad with the steak strips. Drizzle the blue cheese dressing on top of the dish generously and serve.

SESAME BEEF

PREP TIME: 5 MINS | COOK TIME: 5 MINS | SERVES 4

INGREDIENTS:

- Salt (as required)
- ½ tsp. Black pepper (freshly ground)
- 2 tbsp. Sesame oil
- 2 ½ tbsp. Brown sugar
- 3 Garlic cloves (finely chopped)
- 2 Scallions (finely sliced)
- Toasted sesame seeds for garnish (optional)
- 1 lb. Ribeye steak (thinly sliced)

DIRECTIONS:

1. Whisk the sesame oil, soy sauce, garlic, brown sugar, and pepper in a small-sized bowl until the ingredients have blended.
2. Add the ribeye strips in a large-sized bowl, and pour the soy sauce mixture in. Make sure the strips are completely coated in the sauce. Cover the bowl and refrigerate for 60 minutes.
3. Place the grill grate inside the Foodi Grill and secure the hood. Choose the 'GRILL' option and set the timer for 5 minutes at MEDIUM temperature. Press the START/STOP button to allow the unit to preheat.
4. Once the unit beeps and is ready to cook, arrange the beef strips on the grill grate. Close the grill hood and cook for about 4 minutes.
5. Check if the steak is well-cooked after 4 minutes. If required, cook the steak strips for 1 more minute.
6. When the steak strips are cooked, transfer them to a serving plate and garnish with scallions and/or sesame seeds, and serve.

BACON COVERED MEATLOAF

PREP TIME: 5 MINS | COOK TIME: 35 MINS | SERVES 4

INGREDIENTS:

- Salt (as required)
- Black pepper (ground, as required)
- 2 Eggs (large)
- 2 lbs. Beef (ground)
- 8 Slices of bacon
- 1 cup Milk
- 1 tbsp. Worcestershire sauce

- 1 cup bread crumbs
- 2 packs of Onion soup
- ½ Onion (finely chopped)
- 1 cup button mushrooms (diced)
- 4 Garlic cloves (finely chopped)
- 8 oz. Swiss cheese (cubed)
- Olive oil for sautéing

For the Sauce
- ½ cup Mushrooms (chopped)
- 1 cup Chicken broth
- 1 can Cream of mushroom soup
- 1 tsp. Worcestershire sauce
- 2 tbsp. Butter

DIRECTIONS:

1. Sautee the mushrooms and onion in a medium-sized frying pan with Olive oil.
2. Combine all the ingredients (except the beef and bacon) in a large-sized bowl and mix well. Add the sautéed vegetable and beef next. Use your hand to mix the veggies and ground beef with the other ingredients until combined well.
3. Next, place the cooking pot in the Ninja Foodi Grill and secure the hood. Choose the 'GRILL' option and set the timer for 20 minutes at 375°F. Press the START/STOP button to allow the unit to preheat.
4. Load the ground beef into a 9x5-inch meatloaf pan after greasing it. Once the unit beeps and is ready to cook, carefully place the pan in the cooking pot. Secure the lid and cook for 20 minutes.
5. Next, remove the meatloaf pan and cover the top with bacon strips - from end to end. Reduce the temperature to 360°F; place the pan inside the unit, and cook for another 20 minutes.
6. While the meatloaf is cooking, add all the ingredients for the gravy to an adequately-sized frying pan. Cook the gravy for 5 to 6 minutes or until the sauce develops a thick consistency.
7. Once the cooking cycle is complete, and the meatloaf is cooked through, remove the pan from the grill and allow it to rest. After 10 to 15 minutes, cover the meatloaf pan with a serving dish and tilt it 180 degrees. When the meatloaf is on the serving dish, cover it with another plate and tilt once more, so the bacon covered side is facing up.
8. When you're ready, serve a slice of the bacon covered meatloaf with the gravy.

SPICY GRILLED FLANK

PREP TIME: 10 MINS | COOK TIME: 8 MINS | SERVES 2

INGREDIENTS:

- 1 tsp. Sea salt
- ¼ tsp. Black pepper (freshly ground)
- 1 tbsp. Chili powder
- 1 tsp. Thyme (dried)

- 2 tsp. Cumin (ground)
- 2 Flank steaks (8 oz. each)

DIRECTIONS:

1. Place the grill grate inside the Foodi grill and secure the hood. Choose the 'GRILL' option and set the timer for 8 minutes at HIGH temperature. Press the START/STOP to allow the unit to preheat.
2. Mix the thyme, cumin, chili powder, pepper, and salt in a medium-sized bowl. Add the steaks to the spice mixture (one at a time) and use your hand to rub the spices over the meat.
3. When the unit beeps and is heated, arrange the steaks on the grill grate. Press down gently on the steaks to ensure grill marks. Secure the hood and cook for 4 minutes. Open the hood to turn the steaks over and cook for an additional 4 minutes.
4. Once the steaks are done cooking, transfer them to a cutting board to rest for 5 minutes. After 5 minutes, slice the steaks to your preference and serve.

CURRIED LAMB SKEWERS

PREP TIME: 35 MINS | COOK TIME: 45 MINS | SERVES 8

INGREDIENTS:

- 1 ½ tsp. Salt
- 1 tsp. Black pepper (freshly ground)
- 1 tsp. Cumin
- 1 tsp. Red chili powder
- 1 tsp. Garam masala
- 3 Green chilies (de-seeded, minced)
- ¼ Onion (chopped)
- 5 Garlic cloves (minced)
- 10 Coriander stalks (minced)
- 1.4 oz. Lamb (minced)
- 8 Wooden skewers (soaked for 2 to 3 hours)
- Oil for brushing

DIRECTIONS:

1. Toast cumin seeds in a frying pan over medium heat until aromatic. Make sure not to burn the cumin and adjust the heat accordingly. Once done, transfer the cumin to a food processor along with all the other ingredients.
2. Process the ingredients quickly, and make sure not to over mix. You can also mix the ingredients by hand if you prefer.
3. Once the lamb mixture is ready, divide it into 8 equal portions. Lightly wet your hands with cold water, and then squeeze each lamb portion onto the wooden skewers.
4. Transfer the skewers to a plate and refrigerate for 30 minutes. Next, place the grill grate inside the Foodi grill and secure the lid.
5. Choose the 'GRILL' option and set the timer for 12 minutes at MAX temperature. Brush the kebabs with oil and transfer to the grill grate when you hear the unit beep.
6. Secure the grill hood and cook for 6 minutes. Open the hood, turn the skewers, and cook again. At the 10 minute mark, check to see if the lamb isn't browning too fast. Once the cooking cycle is over, transfer the skewers to a serving plate, and serve hot.

JUICY GRILLED FILET WITH SALSA

PREP TIME: 15 MINS | COOK TIME: 8 MINS | SERVES 4

INGREDIENTS:

- Sea salt (as required)
- Black pepper (freshly ground, as required)
- 1 tbsp. Canola oil
- 1 tsp. Chili powder
- ½ tsp. Coriander (ground)
- ½ Pineapple (medium-sized, diced)
- 1 Onion (finely chopped)
- 1 tbsp. Lemon juice (freshly squeezed)
- 2 tbsp. Sliced jalapeño peppers (drained)
- ¼ cup Fresh Cilantro leaves (finely chopped)
- 4 Filet mignon steaks (6-8 oz. each)

DIRECTIONS:

1. Start by rubbing each filet with oil on all sides and season with pepper and salt.
2. Place the grill grate inside the grill and choose the 'GRILL' option. Set the timer for 8 minutes at HIGH temperature. Press the START/STOP button to commence preheating.
3. When the unit beeps and is ready to cook, arrange the filets on the grill grate and secure the hood. Remember to press down on filets to ensure grill marks. Secure the hood and cook for 4 minutes.
4. Once 4 minutes are up, open the grill hood and turn the filets over. Secure the hood again and cook for another 4 minutes. The internal temperature of the filets should read 125°F (at least) on a food thermometer when you take them out of the grill.
5. Allow the filets to rest for 10 minutes at a minimum.
6. In a medium-sized bowl, combine the onions, jalapeños, and diced pineapple. Add cilantro leaves and lime juice. Next, season the salsa with chili powder and ground coriander.
7. Transfer the filets to serving plates and serve with a generous helping of the salsa.

NEW YORK STEAK KEBOBS

PREP TIME: 5 MINS | COOK TIME: 15 MINS | SERVES 4

INGREDIENTS:

- 1/2 cup vegetable oil
- 3 tbsp. Sesame oil
- 1/3 cup Sugar
- 3/4 cup Soy sauce
- 5 Garlic cloves (minced)
- 1 cup whole white mushrooms (quartered)
- 1 Onion (cut into 2-inch cubes)
- 1 Red bell pepper (de-seeded, cut into 2-inch cubes)
- 2 New York strip steaks (10 to 12 oz. each, cut into 2-inch cubes)

DIRECTIONS:

1. In an adequately-sized bowl, add the soy sauce, sesame oil, garlic, vegetable oil, and sugar. Whisk the ingredients until combined. Add the strip steaks to the mixture and use tongs to coat them thoroughly. Cover the bowl and refrigerate for 30 minutes.
2. Place the grill grate inside the Foodi Grill and secure the hood. Choose the 'GRILL' option and set the timer for 12 minutes at MEDIUM temperature. Press the START/STOP button to allow the unit to preheat.
3. Next, assemble the skewers by threading steak, mushroom, bell pepper, and onion cubes. Remember to put the ingredients towards the end of the skewers.
4. Once the unit beeps and is ready to cook, arrange the skewers on the grill grate and secure the hood. Cook the skewers for 8 minutes.
5. Once 8 minutes are up, check to see if the steak cubes are cooked well. If the meat requires more heat, cook for 4 additional minutes.
6. Once the cooking cycle is over, transfer the skewers to a serving plate, and serve hot.

MEATY MARINARA SUB

PREP TIME: 5 MINS | COOK TIME: 10 MINS | SERVES 4

INGREDIENTS:

- Salt (as required)
- Black pepper (freshly ground, as required)
- 1/2 cup Marinara sauce (slightly warmed)
- 8 Mozzarella Slices
- 12 Fresh basil leaves
- 4 Sub rolls (cut in half lengthwise)
- 12 Meatballs (frozen)

DIRECTIONS:

1. Place the crisper basket inside the Ninja Foodi Grill and choose the 'AIR CRISP' option. Set the timer for 10 minutes at 350°F. Press the START/STOP button to allow the unit to preheat.
2. When the unit beeps and is ready to cook, add the meatballs to the crisper basket. Secure the grill hood and cook for 5 minutes.
3. Once 5 minutes are up, take the crisper basket out and give it a shake to make sure the meatballs are evenly cooked. Next, place the basket back into the unit and cook for the remainder of the time.
4. To prepare the subs, add two slices of mozzarella slices on each roll. Spread the marinara sauce generously on top of the cheese and add three basil leaves on top.
5. Once the meatballs are done cooking, place 3 meatballs per roll, and serve hot.

STICKY GINGER RIBS

PREP TIME: 10 MINS | COOK TIME: 25 MINS | SERVES 4

INGREDIENTS:

- 1 tsp. Salt
- 2 tbsp. Vinegar
- 2 tbsp. Sesame oil
- 1 1/2 tbsp. brown sugar
- 1/4 cup Soy sauce
- 1/4 cup Gochujang paste
- 1/4 cup Orange juice (freshly squeezed)
- 6 Garlic cloves (finely chopped)
- 4 Baby back ribs (8 to 10 oz. each)

DIRECTIONS:

1. Add the soy sauce, orange juice, gochujang paste, garlic, sugar, vinegar, oil, and salt in a medium-sized bowl and whisk to combine.
2. Arrange the ribs on a baking sheet and brush with the sauce generously on all sides. Cover the sheet with aluminum foil and refrigerate for 6 hours.
3. Place the grill grate inside the Foodi grill and choose the 'GRILL' option. Set the timer for 22 minutes at MEDIUM temperature. Press the START/STOP button to initiate the preheating process.
4. Once the unit beeps and is ready to cook, arrange the baby back ribs on the grill grate. Secure the grill hood and cook for 11 minutes. Once 11 minutes have passed, flip the ribs over and cook for the remainder of the time.
5. When the cooking cycle has ended, transfer the ribs to a serving plate and serve.

BBQ PORK CHOPS

PREP TIME: 5 MINS | COOK TIME: 35 MINS | SERVES 4

INGREDIENTS:

- Salt (as required)
- Black pepper (freshly ground, as required)
- 1/2 tbsp. Dijon mustard
- 3 tbsp. Worcestershire sauce
- 1 cup Brown sugar (packed)
- 1/4 cup Apple cider vinegar
- 1/4 cup Soy sauce
- 3/4 cup Bourbon
- 2 cups Ketchup
- 4 Pork chops (boneless)

DIRECTIONS:

1. Place a medium-sized saucepan over medium heat, and add the bourbon, vinegar, sugar, ketchup, soy sauce, Worcestershire sauce, and Dijon mustard. Stir the contents together until well combined and bring the mixture to a boil.
2. Next, reduce the heat and allow the sauce mixture to simmer (uncovered). Keep stirring at 20 minutes intervals. Wait until the barbecue sauce develops a thick consistency to remove from the heat.
3. While the barbecue sauce is simmering, place the grill grate inside the Foodi grill and choose the 'GRILL' option. Set the timer for 15 minutes at MEDIUM temperature. Press the START/STOP button to allow the unit to preheat.
4. Once the unit beeps and is ready to cook, arrange the pork chops on the grill grate. Secure the hood and cook the pork for 8 minutes. Once 8 minutes are up, turn the pork chops over and generously coat with barbecue sauce. Close the lid, and cook for an additional 5 minutes.
5. After 5 minutes, open the hood and baste both sides of the pork chops. Remember to flip the pork chops before closing the hood. Continue cooking the pork for the 2 remaining minutes.
6. Once the cooking cycle is over, transfer the pork chops to a serving plate. Season with salt and pepper before serving.

SOY PORK LOIN

PREP TIME: 5 MINS | COOK TIME: 35 MINS | SERVES 4

INGREDIENTS:

- 1/2 tsp. Salt
- 1/2 tsp. Garlic powder
- 1/2 tsp. Onion powder
- 1 tbsp. Soy sauce
- 2 tbsp. Honey
- 1 Pork tenderloin (1 1/2 lbs.)

DIRECTIONS:

1. Place the grill grate inside the Food grill and secure the hood. Choose the 'GRILL' option and set the timer for 20 minutes at MEDIUM temperature. Press the START/STOP button to allow the preheating process to begin.
2. Combine the soy sauce, onion powder, garlic powder, honey, and salt in a small-sized bowl and whisk together.
3. Once you hear the unit beep and Foodi Grill is ready to cook, arrange the pork tenderloin on the grill grate. Make sure to baste the tenderloin of all sides with the soy sauce mixture. Secure the grill lid, and cook for 8 minutes. Once 8 minutes have passed, turn the tenderloin over and baste with sauce again. Continue to cook the meat for 7 minutes.
4. After 15 minutes of cooking time are over, check the internal temperature of the tenderloin. The reading on a food thermometer needs to be at least 145°F. If the temperature reading is lower than that, cook the pork for an additional 5 minutes.
5. When the cooking cycle is over, transfer the tenderloin to a cutting board and allow it to rest for 5 to 10 minutes. After resting, you can slice the tenderloin according to your preference and serve.

KOREAN-STYLE BEEF

PREP TIME: 5 MINS | COOK TIME: 15 MINS | SERVES 4

INGREDIENTS:

- Sea salt (as required)
- 1 tsp. Black pepper (freshly ground)
- 3 tbsp. Brown sugar
- 3 tbsp. Sesame oil
- 1/3 cup Soy sauce
- 4 Garlic cloves (finely chopped)
- 1 tsp. Ginger (finely chopped)
- 1/2 Apple (peeled, shredded)
- 11/2 lbs. Beef tips

DIRECTIONS:

1. Add the apple, sesame oil, sugar, garlic, ginger, pepper, salt, and soy sauce in a medium-sized bowl and mix well.
2. Take a large-sized bowl and add the beef tips and soy sauce mixture to it. Make sure the tips are well coated with the mixture, then cover the bowl and refrigerate for 30 minutes.
3. Place the grill grate inside the Foodi unit and choose the 'GRILL' option. Set the timer for 13 minutes at MEDIUM temperature. Press the START/STOP button to allow the grill unit to preheat.
4. Once the unit beeps and is ready to cook, arrange the beef tips on the grill grate. Secure the hood and cook for 11 minutes.
5. The beef tips will be ready once the internal temperature reads 145°F on a food thermometer. After 11 minutes, check the internal temperature of the steak tips. If the reading on the thermometer is lower than 145°F, then cook for an additional 2 minutes.
6. Once the cooking cycle is over, transfer the steak tips to a cutting board. Allow the meat to rest for 5 minutes and then serve.

SPICY CHEESE BURGERS

PREP TIME: 5 MINS | COOK TIME: 10 MINS | SERVES 4

INGREDIENTS:

- Salt (as required)
- 1/4 tsp. Black pepper (freshly ground)
- 1/4 tsp. Paprika
- 1/2 cup Cheddar (shredded)
- 4 oz. Cream cheese (room temperature)
- 4 Pepper jack slices
- 2 Jalapeño peppers (seeded, tops removed, minced)
- 2 lbs. Beef (ground)
- 4 Bacon sliced (cooked, crumbled)
- 4 Hamburger buns
- Lettuce, tomatoes, onions (sliced, for burger toppings)

DIRECTIONS:

1. Place the grill grate inside the grill unit. Choose the 'GRILL' option and set the timer for 9 minutes at HIGH temperature. Press the START/STOP button to allow the Foodi unit to preheat.
2. Add the cheddar, cream cheese, bacon, and peppers in a medium-sized bowl and mix well.
3. Wet your hands with cold water and form 8 patties (with 8 1/4-inch thickness) with the ground beef. Next, add the cream cheese filling on top of four patties and cover them with the other four. Make sure to pinch the edges of the patty to hold the filling in. If necessary, reshape the burger patties with your hand again.
4. In a small bowl, combine the paprika, salt, and black pepper and mix well. Sprinkle the burger patties with this spice mixture on both sides.
5. Once the unit beeps and is ready to cook, arrange the hamburger patties on the grill grate and secure the hood. Cook the hamburgers for 4 minutes (without turning over). The patties will be ready when their internal temperature reads 145°F (at least) on a food thermometer. Check to see if the temperature of the hamburgers is as required. If not, cook them for an additional 5 minutes.
6. Once the hamburgers are ready, add them to the burger buns. Don't forget to top off with lettuce, tomato, onion, and cheese slices.

ROSEMARY LAMB

PREP TIME: 15 MINS | COOK TIME: 8 MINS | SERVES 4

INGREDIENTS:

- Sea salt (as required)
- 1 tablespoon rosemary(freshly and chopped)
- Black pepper (freshly ground, as required)
- 3 tbsp. Olive oil (extra virgin)
- 1 tbsp. Fresh basil (finely chopped)
- 1 Garlic clove (finely chopped)
- 1/2 Lamb rack (with 4 bones)

DIRECTIONS:

1. In a large-sized bowl, combine the garlic, basil, oil, and mix the ingredients well. Next, flavor the rack of lamb with salt and pepper and place it in the oil mixture bowl. Make sure to coat the lamb with the oil mixture with the use of tongs. Cover the bowl and place it in the fridge for 2 hours.
2. Place the grill grate inside the Foodi grill and choose the 'GRILL' option. Set the timer for 14 minutes at HIGH temperature. Press the START/STOP button to allow the unit to preheat.
3. Once the unit beeps and is ready to cook, arrange the lamb rack on the grill grate and cook for 6 minutes. When 6 minutes are up, open the grill hood to turn the lamb rack over. Continue cooking the meat for another 6 minutes.
4. The lamb will be ready to consume when the internal temperature reads 145°F (at minimum) on a food thermometer. If the reading is lower than what's required, cook the lamb for another 2 minutes.

HOISIN PORK RIBS

PREP TIME: 10 MINS | COOK TIME: 25 MINS | SERVES 2

INGREDIENTS:

- 1 tsp. Black pepper (freshly ground)
- 1 tsp. Garlic powder
- 1 tsp. Onion powder
- 1/4 cup Hoisin sauce
- 1/4 cup Soy sauce
- 1/4 cup Rice vinegar
- 1 lb. Pork ribs

DIRECTIONS:

1. In a large-sized bowl, add all the ingredients (except pork) and mix well.
2. Next, add the pork ribs and turn over several times to coat well in the sauce. Cover the bowl and refrigerate for 2 to 4 hours.
3. Place the grill grate inside the Foodi Grill and choose the 'GRILL' option. Set the timer for 24 minutes at MEDIUM temperature. Press the START/STOP button to allow the unit to preheat.
4. Once the unit beeps and is ready to cook, arrange the pork ribs on the grill grate and secure the grill hood. Cook the pork ribs for 12 minutes.
5. Once 12 minutes are up, open the grill hood and turn the ribs over. Secure the lid and continue cooking for the remainder of the time.
6. Once the cooking cycle is over, transfer the pork ribs to a serving plate and serve.

COLA ROASTED STEAK

PREP TIME: 10 MINS | COOK TIME: 40 MINS | SERVES 4

INGREDIENTS:

- 1 tsp. Salt
- 1 tsp. Black pepper (freshly ground)
- 1 can Cola
- 1/2 cup Water
- 2 Garlic cloves (minced)
- 1 tsp. Thyme
- 2 lbs. Beef sirloin

DIRECTIONS:

1. Place the cooking pot (lightly greased) inside the Foodi Grill and choose the 'ROAST' option. Set the timer for 40 minutes at 400°F. Press the START/STOP button to allow the unit to preheat.
2. Once the unit beeps and is ready to cook, open the grill and add all the ingredients and stir. Place the beef sirloin in at the end. Secure the hood and allow the beef to cook for 40 minutes without interruption.
3. Once the cooking cycle is over, transfer the beef sirloin to a serving plate and serve.

TENDER TOPSIDE ROAST

PREP TIME: 10 MINS | COOK TIME: 30 MINS | SERVES 6

INGREDIENTS:

- Salt (as required)
- Black pepper (ground, as required)
- 1 tbsp. Butter
- 3 tbsp. Olive oil (extra virgin)
- 2 tbsp. Parsley (finely chopped)
- 1 tbsp. Rosemary (finely chopped)
- 1 sprig of Thyme
- 1 Garlic bulb (peeled, crushed)
- 2 Onions (roughly chopped)
- 2 Celery stalks (finely chopped)
- 2 lbs. Topside of beef

DIRECTIONS:

1. In a large-sized bowl, combine all the ingredients and mix well. Make sure the beef and the vegetables are coated with the seasonings.
2. Place the cooking pot (lightly greased with cooking spray) inside the Foodi Grill and secure the hood. Choose the 'ROAST' option and set the timer for 30 minutes at 380°F. Press the START/STOP button to allow the unit to preheat.
3. Once the unit beeps and is ready to cook, add all the ingredients of the bowl to the cooking pot. Close the grill hood and cook for 40 minutes.
4. Once the cooking cycle is completed, transfer the beef to a serving plate, and serve.

PORK TENDERLOIN WITH PEARS

PREP TIME: 10 MINS | COOK TIME: 12 MINS | SERVES 6

INGREDIENTS:

- Salt (as required)
- 1/2 tsp. Black pepper (freshly ground)
- 2 tbsp. Olive oil (extra virgin)
- 1 1/2 tsp. Cumin (ground)
- 1 1/2 tsp. Oregano (dried)
- 1/4 cup lemon juice (fresh squeezed)
- 2 Garlic cloves (finely chopped)
- 2 lbs. Pork tenderloin (3/4-inch thickness)

Pear mix
- 1 tbsp. Lemon zest (grated)
- 1/2 tsp. Black pepper (freshly ground)
- 2 tbsp. Lemon juice
- 1 tbsp. Sugar
- 2 tbsp. Fresh mint (finely chopped)
- 1/3 cup Onions (diced)
- 4 cup Pears (peeled, diced)

- 1 jalapeño pepper (de-seeded, minced)

DIRECTIONS:

1. In a large-sized bowl, add the lemon juice, oregano, oil, cumin, garlic, salt, pepper, and mix the ingredients until well combined. Then add the pork tenderloin to the marinade and coat with the marinade on all sides. Cover the bowl and place in the fridge for 8 hours or overnight.
2. Add the pear mix ingredients in an adequately-sized bowl and mix well. Set the bowl aside for later.
3. Put the grill grate inside the Ninja Foodi Grill and choose the 'GRILL' option. Set the timer for 12 minutes at HIGH temperature. Secure the hood and press the START/STOP button to allow the unit to preheat.
4. Once the unit is ready to cook and beeps to alert you, arrange the pork tenderloin slices on the grill grate and close the grill lid. Allow the cooking cycle to commence.
5. Cook the pork for 6 minutes, then open the hood and turn the pork tenderloin for an even cook. Secure the hood yet again and cook for the remainder of the time.
6. When the timer reads zero, transfer the tenderloin slices to a serving plate and serve with a side of delicious pear mix.

CLASSIC GARLIC GRILLED PORK CHOPS

PREP TIME: 10 MINS | COOK TIME: 15 MINS | SERVES 2

INGREDIENTS:

- 1/2 tsp. Salt
- 1/4 tsp. Sugar
- 1 tbsp. Black pepper (cracked)
- 2 tbsp. Garlic (finely chopped)
- 1 tbsp. Cumin (ground)

- 1 tbsp. Olive oil (extra virgin)
- 2 Pork chops

DIRECTIONS:

1. Add all the ingredients (except the pork chops) to a large-sized bowl and mix well.
2. Next, add the pork chops and coat well with the seasonings. Cover the bowl and place in the refrigerator for 2 to 4 hours.
3. Place the grill grate inside the Foodi Grill and secure the hood. Choose the 'GRILL' option and set the timer for 15 minutes and MEDIUM temperature. Press the START/STOP to commence the preheating process.
4. Once the unit beeps and is ready to cook, arrange the pork chops on the grill grate. Secure the grill hood and cook for 8 minutes.
5. After 8 minutes have passed; turn the pork chops over for an even cook. Cover the lid and cook for the remainder of the time.
6. Once the timer read zero, transfer the pork chops to serving plates and serve.

BEEF ROASTED IN RED WINE

PREP TIME: 10 MINS | COOK TIME: 45 MINS | SERVES 4

INGREDIENTS:

- Salt (as required)
- Black pepper (freshly ground, as required)
- 3/4 cup Red wine vinegar
- 1 Onion (thinly sliced)
- 10 Garlic cloves (finely chopped)
- 1 bunch of Cilantro (finely chopped)
- 3 lbs. Beef brisket

DIRECTIONS:

1. Add the garlic, onions, cilantro, and red wine to a blender and blend to a smooth consistency. Add salt and pepper according to preference.
2. Add the red wine to a large resealable bag, and place the beef brisket inside next. Seal the bag and gently shake to coat the beef briskets with the marinade. Place the bag in the refrigerator for 2 to 4 hours.
3. Place the cooking pot (lightly greased with cooking spray) inside the Foodi Grill and secure the hood. Choose the 'ROAST' option and set the timer for 45 minutes at 350°F. Press the START/STOP button to allow the unit to preheat.
4. Once the unit beeps and is heated, add the beef brisket to the cooking pot and secure the grill hood.
5. Cook the briskets for 45 minutes without interruptions. Serve the beef briskets warm when ready.

RICOTTA TENDERLOIN PASTA

PREP TIME: 10 MINS | COOK TIME: 15 MINS | SERVES 4

INGREDIENTS:

- 1/2 tsp. Salt
- 1/2 tsp. Black pepper (freshly ground)
- 1/2 cup Walnuts (roughly chopped)
- 1/2 cup Ricotta (crumbled)
- 2/3 cup Pesto
- 4 cups Grape tomatoes (halved)
- 10 oz. Baby spinach (roughly chopped)
- 4 cups Penne pasta (uncooked)
- 4 Beef tenderloin steaks (6 oz. each)

DIRECTIONS:

1. Start by cooking the penne pasta (as directed on its pack) in water seasoned with salt. Drain the pasta when done and set aside for later.
2. Place the beef tenderloin steaks on a clean work surface and season with pepper and salt on all sides.
3. Place the grill grate in the Foodi Grill and choose the 'GRILL' option. Secure the hood, and set the timer for 14 minutes at HIGH temperature. Press the START/STOP button to start the preheating process.
4. Once the unit beeps and is heated, arrange the beef steaks on the grill grate and close the hood. Let the beef cook for 7 minutes.
5. Once 7 minutes are over, open the grill hood and turn the steaks for an even cook. Then proceed to cook for the remainder of the cooking time.
6. In a large-sized bowl, add the tomatoes, walnuts, pesto, spinach, pasta, and mix until the ingredients are well combined.
7. When the steaks are cooked, transfer them to a cutting board to rest. After 5 minutes, arrange the steaks on a serving plate with a side of the pesto salad, topped with ricotta.

CRUMBED PORK CHOPS

PREP TIME: 10 MINS | COOK TIME: 25 MINS | SERVES 4

INGREDIENTS:

- Salt (as required)
- Black pepper (freshly ground, as required)
- 1 Egg
- 1/2 tsp. Garlic powder
- 1/2 tsp. Cayenne pepper
- 1/2 tsp. Dijon mustard

- 4 tsp. Paprika
- 1/4 cup Milk
- 1 cup Panko breadcrumbs
- 4 Pork chops (bone-in)

DIRECTIONS:

1. Prepare the pork tenderloins by seasoning with salt and pepper on all sides.
2. In a small bowl, add the milk and egg. Whisk until well combined.
3. Add the garlic powder, paprika, cayenne pepper, Dijon mustard, breadcrumbs, and mix well.
4. Dip the pork tenderloins with the egg mixture and then dip into the breadcrumbs to form a coat.
5. Place the crisper basket inside the Foodi grill and secure the grill hood. Choose the 'AIR CRISP' option and set the timer for 25 minutes at 400°F. Press the START/STOP button to start the preheating process.
6. When the unit beeps and is ready to cook, arrange the pork tenderloins inside the crisper basket. Secure the hood and cook for 25 minutes.
7. Once the cooking cycle is complete, transfer the pork tenderloins to a serving plate and enjoy.

SAVORY SAUSAGE PASTRY

PREP TIME: 15 MINS | COOK TIME: 45 MINS | SERVES 6

INGREDIENTS:

- Salt (as required)
- Black pepper (as required)
- 2 tbsp. Caramelized onion chutney
- 1 tbsp. Fresh basil (finely chopped)
- 1 Egg (whisked for glazing pastry)

- 9 oz. pack of Puff pastry
- 14 oz. Pork sausage meat

DIRECTIONS:

1. Place the cooking pot (lightly greased) in the Foodi Grill unit and choose the 'BAKE' option. Set the timer for 30 minutes at 320°F. Press the START/STOP button to start the preheating process.
2. Add the chutney, basil, salt, pepper, and sausage meat in a large-sized bowl and mix. Once the ingredients are well combined, make a thick sausage from the mixture (at least 8.5 inches long)
3. Line the Ninja Foodi crisper basket with baking parchment and set aside. Dust flour on a flat work surface and roll the puff pastry into a rectangular shape measuring 9.5x11 inches. Carefully transfer the rolled out pastry to the crisper basket and place the sausage in the middle (leave a 1-inch gap on all sides).
4. Make diagonal cuts (with 2-inch gaps) along the length of the pastry. Fold the ends to form a pastry plait on top of the sausage. Trim any excess pastry. Lightly brush the pastry surface with the egg mixture.
5. Once the unit beeps and is ready to cook, place the crisper basket in the cooking pot, and secure the hood. Cook the pastry for 30 minutes.
6. When the cooking cycle is complete, carefully transfer the pastry to a cutting board and cool for 5 minutes. When you're ready, serve the sausage plait hot or cold.

SEAFOOD

PARMESAN SHRIMP SALAD

PREP TIME: 10 MINS | COOK TIME: 5 MINS | SERVES 4

INGREDIENTS:

- Sea salt (as required)
- Black pepper (freshly ground, as required)
- Juice of ½ a lime (freshly squeezed)
- 2 Romaine lettuce heads (roughly chopped)
- 3 Garlic cloves (finely chopped)
- ½ cup Parmesan cheese (shredded))
- ¾ cup Caesar dressing
- 1 lb. Jumbo shrimp (fresh)

DIRECTIONS:

1. Place the grill grate inside the Foodi grill unit and secure the hood. Choose the 'GRILL' option and set the timer for 5 minutes at MAX temperature. Press the START/STOP button to commence the preheating process.
2. Toss the shrimp in lime juice, salt, black pepper, and garlic in a large-sized bowl. Let the shrimps marinate.
3. The Foodi unit will be ready for cooking once it beeps. Open the grill hood and arrange the shrimps on the grill grate. Close the lid and allow the shrimp to cook for 5 minutes.
4. Next, in an adequately-sized bowl, toss the lettuce with the Caesar dressing. Then divide and place the lettuce on four separate serving plates.
5. Once the shrimp is cooked, use tongs to transfer the shrimps onto the serving plates. Place the meat on top of the salad, and sprinkle generously with parmesan cheese to serve.

GARLIC & CHILI PRAWNS

PREP TIME: 5 MINS | COOK TIME: 20 MINS | SERVES 4

INGREDIENTS:

- Sea salt (as required)
- 7 tbsp. Olive oil (extra virgin)
- ½ tsp. Sweet paprika powder
- ½ tsp. Red pepper flakes
- 8 Garlic cloves (minced)
- Juice of ½ lemon (freshly squeezed)
- 20 Large king prawns (head removed, deveined)

DIRECTIONS:

1. Place the air fryer basket inside the Foodi Grill and secure the hood. Choose the 'AIR FRY' option and set the timer for 5 minutes at 248°F. Press the START/STOP button to allow the grill to preheat.
2. Once the unit is ready to cook and beeps, arrange the prawns on the basket and cook for 5 minutes. Remember to turn the prawns at the halfway mark.
3. Next, put a medium-sized pan over high heat, and add olive oil. Once the oil is ready, add the red pepper flakes and garlic. Cook the oil for 3 minutes before adding the prawns. Add the sweet paprika powder, stir the prawns, and take the pan off the heat.
4. Transfer the prawns (with the chili and garlic oil) and serve with a dash of freshly squeezed lemon juice.

SPICED SALMON WITH TAMARIND

PREP TIME: 5 MINS | COOK TIME: 15 MINS | SERVES 3

INGREDIENTS:

- ½ tsp. Salt
- 1 tsp. Cumin (ground)
- ¼ tsp. Turmeric (ground)
- ½ tsp. Red chili powder
- ½ tbsp. Tamarind paste
- 2 tbsp. Olive oil (extra virgin)
- 1 tbsp. Brown sugar (soft)
- 4 Garlic cloves (minced)
- 3 Salmon fillets (7 oz. each)

DIRECTIONS:

1. In a large resealable bag, mix all the ingredients (except the fillets) to create a marinade. Add the salmon fillets to the marinade, seal the bag, and gently shake it to coat the fillets. Place the bag inside the refrigerator for 1 hour.
2. Place the grill plate inside the Foodi Grill and secure the hood. Choose the 'AIR FRY' option and set the timer for 12 minutes at HIGH temperature. Press the START/STOP button to allow the grill to preheat.
3. Once the unit beeps and is ready to cook, arrange the fillets on the grate and cook for 6 minutes.
4. Open the grill hood to check if the salmon is cooking too fast. If the temperature is too high, lower it, and allow the salmon to cook for the remaining time or until it's cooked to your preference.
5. Once the salmon fillets are cooked, transfer them to serving plates, and serve

SOUTHWEST SHRIMP TACOS

PREP TIME: 15 MINS | COOK TIME: 10 MINS | SERVES 4

INGREDIENTS:

- Cooking spray
- 1 tsp. Cumin (ground)
- 1 tsp. Chili powder
- 1 tsp. Southwestern seasoning
- Juice of ½ a lemon (freshly squeezed)
- 1 Avocado (peeled, sliced)
- 2 cups Green cabbage (shredded)
- 1 lb. Jumbo shrimp (fresh)
- 4 Corn tortillas

DIRECTIONS:

1. Place the grill grate inside the Foodi grill unit and secure the hood. Choose the 'GRILL' option and set the timer for 10 minutes at MAX temperature. Press the START/STOP button to start the preheating process.
2. Next, spray both sides of the tortillas with cooking spray and set aside. In a large-sized bowl, toss the shrimp with cumin, chili powder, southwestern seasoning, and lemon juice. Leave the shrimp in the bowl to marinate.
3. Once the unit beeps and is ready to cook, open the grill hood and place a single tortilla on the grate. Secure the hood and allow the tortilla to cook for 1 minute. After one minute, remove the tortilla, and set aside. Repeat the process for the remaining tortillas.
4. Once all the tortillas are cooked, arrange the shrimp on the grill grate, secure the hood and cook for 5 minutes.
5. Once the cooking cycle is complete, remove the shrimp from the grill. On an adequately-sized serving plate, arrange the tortillas and fill with shrimp, avocado, and cabbage. You can also choose to add other ingredients such as feta cheese, cilantro, etc.

ASIAN STYLE COD

PREP TIME: 5 MINS | COOK TIME: 17 MINS | SERVES 4

INGREDIENTS:

- ¼ tsp. Red pepper flakes
- 3 tbsp. Brown sugar
- 1 tsp. Sesame oil (divided as per directions)
- 2 tbsp. Soy sauce
- 1 tbsp. White wine vinegar
- ¼ cup Miso
- 1 lb. Baby bok choy (cut lengthwise down the middle)
- 4 Cod fillets (6 oz. each)

DIRECTIONS:

1. Use a resealable plastic to combine a marinade of brown sugar, miso, and 1/3 tsp. sesame oil. Add the cod to marinade, seal the bag, shake it gently to the fish with the sauce. Put the bad in the refrigerator for 30 minutes.
2. Place the grill grate inside the Foodi unit and secure the hood. Choose the 'GRILL' option and set the timer for 8 minutes at MAX temperature. Press the START/STOP button to start the preheating cycle.
3. Once the unit beeps and is ready to cook, arrange the fillets on the grill grate. Remember to press down on the cod fillets to maximize grill marks. Secure the grill hood and cook for 8 minutes.
4. Add 1/3 tsp. sesame oil, red pepper flakes, and soy sauce in a small-sized bowl. Whisk the ingredients together until they're well combined. Use the soy sauce mixture to brush the bok choy halves from all sides.
5. Once 8 minutes are up, transfer the fillets to a plate or cutting board and cover lightly with aluminum foil.
6. Secure the grill hood again, and choose the 'GRILL' option. Set the timer for 9 minutes at MAX temperature. Press the START/STOP to preheat the grill.
7. Once the unit is ready, open the hood and arrange the bok choy halves on the grill grate. Secure the hood and cook for 9 minutes.
8. Once the bok choy is ready, transfer it to serving plates along with the cod fillets and serve immediately.

GRILLED MAHI MAHI WITH CAPER SAUCE

PREP TIME: 5 MINS | COOK TIME: 8 MINS | SERVES 4

INGREDIENTS:

- Sea salt (as required)
- Black pepper (freshly ground as required)
- 4 tbsp. Butter (unsalted)
- 1 tbsp. Olive oil (extra virgin)
- 1 tbsp. Lemon juice (freshly squeezed)
- 2 tbsp. Green Olives (sliced, drained)
- 2 tbsp. Capers (drained)
- 1 Lemon (cut into 8 equal slices)
- 4 Fresh mahi mahi steaks (with 1-inch thickness)

DIRECTIONS:

1. Whisk the lemon juice and olive oil in a large-sized bowl. Next, season the steaks with salt and pepper (on each side) and place them in the lemon juice mixture. Turn the steaks for an even coat. Place the bowl in the refrigerator for 15 minutes.
2. Place the grill grate inside the grill unit and choose the 'GRILL' option. Set the timer for 8 minutes at MAX temperature, and press the START/STOP button to allow the grill to preheat.
3. Once the unit beeps and is ready to cook, arrange the mahi mahi steaks on the grill grate. Secure the hood and allow the fish to cook for 9 minutes.
4. Proceed to melt the butter in a small-sized saucepan over medium flame. Cook and stir for 3 minutes or until the butter turns light brown. Next, add the olives, capers, and lemon juice to the butter and cook for 1 minute. Take the pan off the heat.
5. Transfer the mahi mahi steaks to serving plates when they're done. Drizzle the steaks with the olive and caper sauce generously and serve.

HONEY-SOY SALMON

PREP TIME: 10 MINS | COOK TIME: 8 MINS | SERVES 4

INGREDIENTS:

- Sea salt (as required)
- Black pepper (freshly ground, as required)
- Zest of ½ Lime
- Juice of 3 limes (divided as per directions)
- 1 tbsp. Olive oil (extra virgin)
- 2 tbsp. Butter (unsalted, melted)
- 1 tbsp. Fish sauce
- 1/3 cup Honey
- 3 Garlic cloves (finely chopped, divided as per directions)
- 1 Mango (peeled, roughly chopped)
- 1 Avocado (peeled, roughly chopped)
- ½ Onion (diced)
- ½ Tomato (diced)
- 1 Jalapeño (de-seeded, finely chopped)
- 4 Skinless salmon fillets (6 oz. each)

DIRECTIONS:

1. Prepare the marinade in a large-sized resealable bag by adding fish sauce, butter, lime zest, honey, 2 minced garlic cloves, and the juice of 2 limes. Add the salmon fillets, seal the bag, and gently shake to coat the fillets in the marinade. Place in the refrigerator for 30 minutes.
2. Next, in a large-sized bowl, combine the avocado, tomato, mango, onion, 1 minced garlic clove, juice of 1 lime, jalapeño, olive oil, pepper, and salt. Gently mix the ingredients, cover the bowl, and refrigerate.
3. Place the grill grate inside the Foodi grill, secure the hood, and set the timer for 8 minutes at MAX temperature. Press the START/STOP button to allow the unit to preheat.
4. Once the unit beeps and is preheated, arrange the salmon fillets on the grill grate. Press down on the fillets gently to ensure grill marks. Secure the grill hood, and allow the salmon to cook for 6 minutes.
5. After 6 minutes, open the hood and check the salmon's temperature. The internal temperature should be at least 140°F on a food thermometer. If the reading is low, close the lid and cook the fillets for another 2 minutes.
6. When the cooking cycle is complete, transfer the fillets to a serving plate and serve immediately with the pre-prepared salsa.

CREAMY SRIRACHA SALMON

PREP TIME: 10 MINS | COOK TIME: 8 MINS | SERVES 4

INGREDIENTS:

- ¼ cup Honey
- 1 cup Sriracha
- Juice of 2 Limes
- Fresh Chives (minced, for garnishing)
- 4 Skinless salmon fillets (6 oz. each)

DIRECTIONS:

1. Prepare the salmon marinade in a resealable bag by adding lemon juice, honey, and sriracha sauce. Place the salmon fillets inside the bag, seal it, and shake gently to coat the fillets with the marinade. Place in the refrigerator for 30 minutes.
2. Place the grill grate inside the unit and secure the grill hood. Choose the 'GRILL' option and set the timer for 8 minutes at MAX temperature. Press the START/STOP button to allow the grill to preheat.
3. Once the unit beeps and is ready to cook, arrange the fillets on the grill grate and gently press down to ensure grill marks. Secure the hood, and allow the fillets to cook for 6 minutes.
4. When 6 minutes are up, open the grill to check the temperature of the fillets. If the reading on a food thermometer is lower than 140°F, then cook the fillet for another 2 minutes.
5. Once 2 minutes have elapsed, transfer the salmon fillets to serving plates. Garnish with fresh chives and serve.

SESAME TUNA WITH BABY GREENS

PREP TIME: 10 MINS | COOK TIME: 6 MINS | SERVES 4

INGREDIENTS:

- ¼ tsp. Salt (plus for seasoning)
- ½ tsp. Black pepper (plus for seasoning)
- 6 tbsp. Canola oil
- 2 tbsp. Sesame oil
- 2 tbsp. White wine vinegar (or rice wine vinegar)
- ½ Cucumber (thinly sliced)
- 10 oz. pack of Baby greens
- 1 ½ lbs. Ahi tuna (cut into four equal strips)

DIRECTIONS:

1. Place the grill grate inside the Foodi grill and secure the hood. Set the timer for 6 minutes at MAX temperature. Press the START/STOP button to initiate the preheating process.
2. Add the canola oil, white wine vinegar, 1/2 tsp. of black pepper, and 1/4 tsp. of salt in a small-sized bowl. Briskly whisk the contents until the ingredients have combined.
3. Next, season the tuna meat with salt and pepper. Finally, drizzle the strips with sesame oil.
4. Once the unit beeps and is ready to cook, arrange the tuna on the grill grate. Close the lid and allow the tuna to cook for 6 minutes.
5. Place equal portions of baby greens and cucumber slices on four serving plates while the tuna is cooking.
6. Once the tuna is ready, place each strip on top of the salad, generously drizzle with the white wine vinaigrette and serve.

HOT & SAUCY FISH SANDWICH

PREP TIME: 10 MINS. | COOK TIME: 15 MINS. | SERVES 4

INGREDIENTS:

- 2 large eggs
- 10 ounces beer
- 1½ teaspoons hot sauce
- 1½ cups cornstarch
- 1½ cups all-purpose flour
- 1 teaspoon of sea salt
- 1 teaspoon ground black pepper
- 4 (6-ounce) cod fillets
- Nonstick cooking spray
- 4 soft rolls, sliced
- Tartar sauce
- Lettuce leaves
- Lemon wedges

DIRECTIONS:

1. Place the Crisper Basket inside the Ninja Foodi Grill and close its hood.
2. Select AIR CRISP mode, set the temperature to 375°F, and cooking time to 15 minutes. Hit the START/STOP button to initiate preheating.
3. Meanwhile, whisk eggs with hot sauce and beer in a large shallow bowl.
4. Whisk cornstarch with flour, salt, and black pepper in another large bowl.
5. Take one cod fillet at a time and dip in the egg mixture, then coat it with the flour mixture. Coat the remaining cod fillets in the same manner.
6. When the unit is preheated, grease its Crisper Basket with the cooking spray.
7. Set the coated fish fillets in the Crisper basket and coat them with cooking spray.
8. Close the hood again and let the fish cook for 15 minutes.
9. Once the fish is done, check the crispiness of the fish, then remove it from the basket.
10. Place one half of each soft roll on a working surface and top it with a layer of tartar sauce.
11. Add one fish fillet and a lettuce leaf on top of the tartar sauce then cover each with the other half of the roll.
12. Serve warm with lemon wedges.

CAJUN CRAB CAKES

PREP TIME: 10 MINS. | COOK TIME: 10 MINS. | SERVES 4

INGREDIENTS:

- 1 egg
- 1/2 cup 3 tablespoons mayonnaise, divided
- Juice of ½ lemon
- 1 tablespoon scallions, minced (green parts)
- 1 teaspoon Old Bay seasoning
- 8 ounces lump crab meat
- 1/3 cup bread crumbs
- Nonstick cooking spray

- 1/2 teaspoon cayenne pepper
- 1/4 teaspoon paprika
- 1/4 teaspoon garlic powder
- 1/4 teaspoon chili powder
- 1/4 teaspoon onion powder
- 1/4 teaspoon ground black pepper
- 1/8 teaspoon ground nutmeg

DIRECTIONS:

1. Place the Crisper Basket inside the Ninja Foodi Grill and close its hood.
2. Select AIR CRISP mode, set the temperature to 375°F, and cooking time to 10 minutes. Hit the START/STOP button to initiate preheating.
3. Meanwhile, beat egg with scallions, lemon juice, Old bay seasoning, and 3 tablespoons mayonnaise in a large bowl.
4. Stir in crabmeat and crumble it into pieces while mixing. Add breadcrumbs and mix well.
5. Divide the mixture into four portions and shape each portion into a patty.
6. Once the unit is preheated, place the crab cakes in the crisper basket and coat them with cooking spray.
7. Close its hood again and let the crab cakes cook for 10 minutes.
8. Meanwhile, whisk ½ cup mayonnaise, paprika, cayenne pepper, chili powder, garlic powder, onion powder, nutmeg, and black pepper in a bowl.
9. Serve the crispy crab cakes with Cajun aioli and devour!

CITRUS SEASONED HALIBUT

PREP TIME: 20 MINS | COOK TIME: 22 MINS | SERVES 4

INGREDIENTS:

- 1 tsp. Salt
- ¼ tsp. Red pepper flakes
- 2 tbsp. Olive oil (extra virgin)
- 2 tbsp. Honey
- 1 tbsp. Ginger (finely chopped)

- 1 tbsp. Garlic (finely chopped)
- 1 tbsp. Fresh chives (finely chopped)
- Juice of 1 lime
- Juice of 1 Orange
- 2 Frozen halibut fillets

DIRECTIONS:

1. Place the grill grate inside the Ninja Foodi Grill and secure the hood. Choose the 'GRILL' option and set the timer for 12 minutes at MAX temperature. Press the START/STOP button to allow the unit to preheat.
2. In a large-sized bowl, combine all the ingredients (except the halibut) and whisk to combine the ingredients well. Next, place the halibut fillets in the bowl. Turn the fillets to coat both sides.
3. When the unit beeps and is ready to begin cooking, set the halibut fillets on the grill grate, and pour a tablespoon of the marinade over each fillet. Secure the grill hood and allow the halibut to cook for 12 minutes or until the internal temperature of the fillets is 149°F. To ensure a strong infusion of citrus flavor, baste the fillets once every 4 minutes.
4. Once the halibut fillets are cooked, transfer to a serving plate, and serve.

GRILLED FRESH GINGER SALMON

PREP TIME: 10 MINS. | COOK TIME: 8 MINS. | SERVES 4

INGREDIENTS:

- ½ tablespoon lime zest, grated
- 1 tablespoon olive oil
- 1/4 teaspoon salt
- 1 tablespoon rice vinegar
- 2 teaspoons sugar
- 1/8 cup lime juice
- 1 cucumber, peeled and chopped

- 1/6 cup cilantro, chopped
- 1 garlic clove, minced
- ½ tablespoon onion, finely chopped
- 1 teaspoon ginger root, minced
- 1/4 teaspoon ground coriander
- 1/4 teaspoon ground pepper

Salmon:
- 1/2 tablespoon olive oil
- 1/6 cup ginger root, minced
- 1/4 teaspoon ground black pepper
- ½ tablespoon lime juice
- 1/4 teaspoon salt
- 5 (6 ounces) salmon fillets

DIRECTIONS:

1. Add lime zest, olive oil, ginger root, ground pepper, lime juice, salt, cilantro, coriander, cucumber, garlic, onion, sugar, and rice vinegar to a food processor.
2. Press the pulse button to puree the mixture into a smooth sauce.
3. Season the salmon fillets by rubbing it with a mixture of lime juice, black pepper, salt, oil, and ginger.
4. Place the grill grate inside the Ninja Foodi Grill and close its hood.
5. Select the "GRILL" mode on the "MED" grill function, set the timer to 8 minutes, then hit the "START/STOP" button to initiate preheating.
6. Once the unit is preheated, place the seasoned salmon fillets in the grill and cover its hood.
7. Let the salmon cook for 4 minutes, then flip its fillets and cover again.
8. Continue cooking the salmon fillets for another 4 minutes.
9. Serve the grilled salmon with the prepared cucumber sauce.

CRUMBED SWEET CHILI PRAWNS

PREP TIME: 15 MINS. | COOK TIME: 14 MINS. | SERVES 4

INGREDIENTS:

- 2 teaspoons ground black pepper
- ½ teaspoon of sea salt
- ½ cup all-purpose flour
- 2 large eggs
- ¾ cup unsweetened coconut flakes
- ¼ cup panko bread crumbs
- 24 prawns, peeled, deveined

- Sweet chili sauce, for serving
- Nonstick cooking spray

DIRECTIONS:

1. Place the Crisper Basket inside the Ninja Foodi Grill and close its hood.
2. Select AIR CRISP mode, set the temperature to 400°F, and cooking time to 7 minutes. Hit the START/STOP button to initiate preheating.
3. Meanwhile, mix flour, salt, and black pepper in a shallow bowl.
4. Beat eggs in one bowl and mix bread crumbs and coconut flakes in another shallow bowl.
5. Coat the prawns with flour mixture, shake off the excess, then dip in the egg and coat with the coconut mixture.
6. Once the unit is preheated, spread half of the coated prawns in the crisper basket and coat them with cooking spray.
7. Close its hood again and let the shrimp cook for 7 minutes.
8. Transfer the cooked prawns to a serving plate and cook the remaining shrimp in the Ninja foodi grill in the same way for 7 minutes.
9. Serve the crispy prawns with sweet chili sauce.

DIJON FISH STICKS

PREP TIME: 10 MINS. | COOK TIME: 10 MINS. | SERVES 4

INGREDIENTS:

- 1-pound cod fillets
- ¼ cup all-purpose flour
- 1 large egg
- ½ cup bread crumbs
- 1 teaspoon Dijon mustard
- 1 tablespoon dried parsley
- 1 teaspoon paprika
- ½ teaspoon ground black pepper
- Nonstick cooking spray

DIRECTIONS:

1. Place the Crisper Basket inside the Ninja Foodi Grill and close its hood.
2. Select AIR CRISP mode, set the temperature to 390°F, and cooking time to 10 minutes. Hit the START/STOP button to initiate preheating.
3. Meanwhile, slice the fish fillets into 1-inch wide sticks and keep them aside.
4. Spread flour on a plate and beat egg with Dijon mustard in a shallow bowl.
5. Mix breadcrumbs with black pepper, paprika, and dried parsley in another shallow bowl.
6. Take one fish stick at a time, coat each of them with flour, dip in the egg, and then coat the fish sticks with the breadcrumb mixture.
7. Once the unit is preheated, place the coated fish sticks in the crisper basket and coat them with cooking spray.
8. Close the hood again and let the fish sticks cook for 10 minutes.
9. Serve warm.

LEMON - GARLIC SHRIMP SKEWERS

PREP TIME: 10 MINS. | COOK TIME: 4 MINS. | SERVES 4

INGREDIENTS:

- 1/3 cup lemon juice
- 2/3 cup fresh arugula
- 1/4 cup yogurt
- 2 teaspoons milk
- 2 tablespoons canola oil
- 1-pound shrimp, peeled and deveined
- 2 green onions, sliced
- 1/2 teaspoon salt
- 1/4 teaspoon ground black pepper
- 1 teaspoon Dijon mustard
- 2 garlic cloves, minced
- 1/2 teaspoon lemon zest, grated
- 1 teaspoon cider vinegar
- 1/2 teaspoon sugar
- 12 cherry tomatoes

DIRECTIONS:

1. Toss shrimp with garlic, oil, lemon zest, and juice in a mixing bowl and leave it for 15 minutes.
2. Meanwhile, blend arugula with green onion, milk, yogurt, vinegar, sugar, ¼ tsp salt, and mustard in a blender until smooth.
3. Thread the shrimp and cherry tomatoes alternately on the wooden skewers (thread 3 shrimp and 3 tomatoes on each skewer).
4. Drizzle black pepper and salt over the shrimp and tomato skewers.
5. Place the grill grate inside the Ninja Foodi Grill and close its hood.
6. Select the "GRILL" mode on the "MED" grill function, set the timer to 4 minutes, then hit the "START/STOP" button to initiate preheating.
7. Once the unit is preheated, place the skewers in the grill and close its hood.
8. Cook the shrimp skewers for 2 minutes, then flip and cook for another 2 minutes.
9. Serve the shrimp skewers with arugula yogurt sauce.

KALAMATA TAPENADE GRILLED SWORDFISH

PREP TIME: 14 MINS. | COOK TIME: 5 MINS. | SERVES 6

INGREDIENTS:

- ½ cup fresh parsley, finely chopped
- ½ tsp dried oregano
- 1 tbsp. lemon juice
- 2 tbsp. canola oil
- 1/8 tsp salt
- 1/3 cup Kalamata olive, pitted and chopped
- ¼ cup celery, finely chopped
- 1 small garlic clove, minced
- Freshly ground black pepper, to taste
- 1¾ pounds swordfish steak, trimmed and cut into 6 pieces
- ¼ tsp salt
- 1/8 tsp ground black pepper
- Lemon wedges, for garnish

DIRECTIONS:

1. Mix olives, parsley, celery, garlic, oregano, lemon juice, salt, black pepper, and 1 tbsp. canola oil in a small bowl.
2. Place the grill grate inside the Ninja Foodi Grill and close its hood.
3. Select the "GRILL" mode on the "Low" grill function, set the timer to 5 minutes, then hit the "START/STOP" button to initiate preheating.
4. Rub the swordfish with 1 tbsp. canola oil, black pepper, and salt for seasoning.
5. Once the unit is preheated, place the steaks in the grill and close its hood.
6. Let the tuna cook for 5 minutes, then transfer it to a serving plate.
7. Garnish with olive relish and lemon wedges.
8. Serve warm.

CRUMBED HADDOCK

PREP TIME: 10 MINS. | COOK TIME: 13 MINS. | SERVES 4

INGREDIENTS:

- 1/4 teaspoons salt
- 3/4 cup breadcrumbs
- 1/4 cup Parmesan cheese, grated
- 1/4 tsp ground dried thyme
- 1/4 cup butter, melted
- 1-pound haddock fillets
- 3/4 cup milk

DIRECTIONS:

1. Mix breadcrumbs with thyme and parmesan cheese in a bowl.
2. First, dip the fish fillets in milk, season them with salt then coat them with the breadcrumb mixture.
3. Select the "Bake" mode on your Ninja Foodi Grill, set the temperature to 325°F and cooking time to 5 minutes, then hit the "START/STOP" button to initiate preheating.
4. Once the unit is preheated, place the coated fish fillets in the grill and close its hood.
5. Let the fish bake for 5 minutes, then flip the fillets and continue cooking for another 8 minutes.
6. Serve warm.

HERB-GRILLED RAINBOW TROUT

PREP TIME: 10 MINS. | COOK TIME: 8 MINS. | SERVES 4

INGREDIENTS:

- 1 tbsp. Canola oil
- 2 cloves of garlic, minced
- 1 tsp dried basil
- 1 tsp ground black pepper
- 1/2 tsp salt
- 1 tbsp. parsley, chopped
- 1 tbsp. lemon juice
- 1-pound rainbow trout fillet

DIRECTIONS:

1. Mix oil, dried basil, garlic, black pepper, salt, parsley, and lemon juice in a shallow bowl.
2. Place the trout fillets in the prepared marinade, rub it over the fish, and cover to refrigerate for 1 hour.
3. Place the grill grate inside the Ninja Foodi grill and close its hood.
4. Select the "Roast" mode, set the temperature to 400°F, and cooking time to 8 minutes, then hit the "START/STOP" button to initiate preheating.
5. Once preheated, place the marinated fillets in the grill, drizzle 1 tbsp. Canola oil, and remaining marinade on top and close the hood.
6. Allow the fish fillets to cook for 8 minutes in the Ninja grill.
7. Serve warm.

SPICY SHRIMP OH' BOY

PREP TIME: 10 MINS. | COOK TIME: 5 MINS. | SERVES 4

INGREDIENTS:

- 2 cups red cabbage, finely shredded
- 2 tbsp. dill pickle relish
- 1-pound raw shrimp, peeled and deveined
- 2 tsp canola oil
- 2 tbsp. mayonnaise
- 2 tbsp. plain yogurt
- 1 tsp chili powder
- ½ tsp paprika
- 4 tomato slices, halved
- ¼ cup red onion, thinly sliced
- ¼ tsp ground black pepper
- 4 whole-wheat hot dog buns split in half

DIRECTIONS:

1. Place the grill grate inside the Ninja Foodi Grill and close its hood.
2. Select the "Grill" mode on the "LOW" grill function and set the timer to 5 minutes, then hit the "START/STOP" button to initiate preheating.
3. Meanwhile, mix yogurt, mayonnaise relish, and cabbage in a medium-sized bowl.
4. Season shrimp by mixing them with black pepper, chili powder, paprika, and 2 tsp oil in a bowl.
5. Place the shrimp in the grill, close its hood, and cook for 5 minutes.
6. Divide the tomato slices, onion, cabbage mixture, and grilled shrimp in the buns.
7. Serve warm.

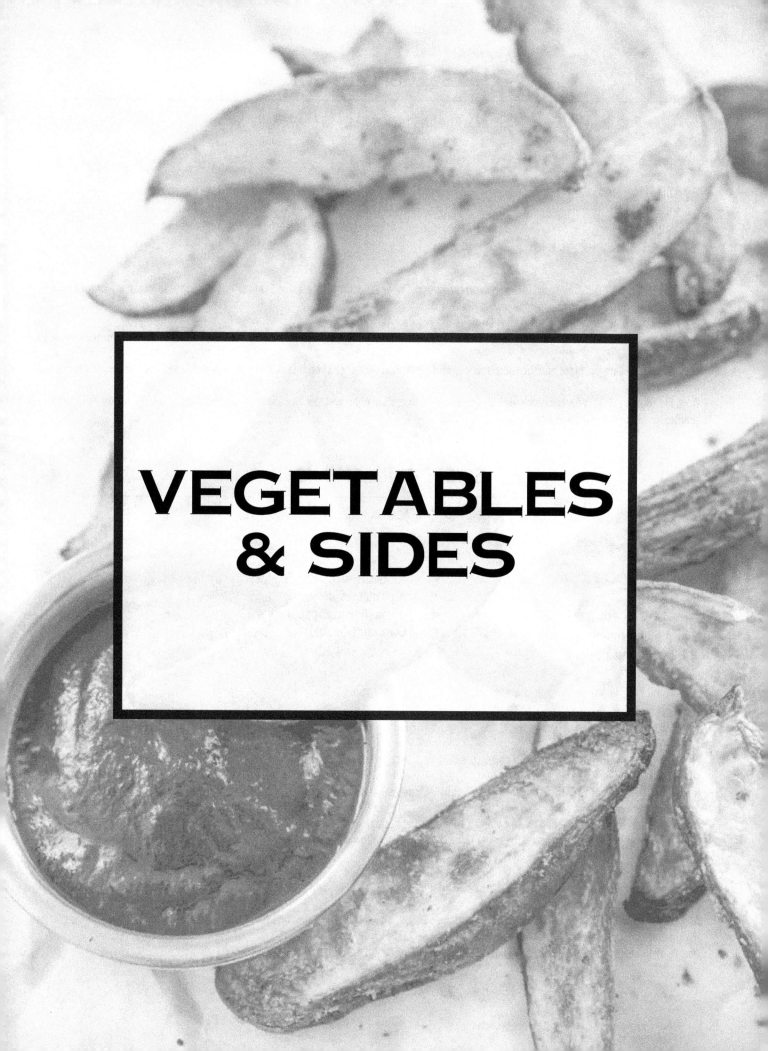

VEGETABLES & SIDES

CHEESY EGGPLANT STACKS

PREP TIME: 10 MINS | COOK TIME: 15 MINS | SERVES 4

INGREDIENTS:

- Sea salt (as required)
- 2 tbsp. Canola oil
- 12 Cilantro leaves
- 1/2 lb. Buffalo mozzarella (sliced with 1/4-inch thickness)
- 1 Eggplant (sliced with 1/4-inch thickness)
- 2 Heirloom tomatoes (sliced with 1/4-inch thickness)

DIRECTIONS:

1. Place the grill grate inside the Foodi Grill and secure the hood. Choose the 'GRILL' option and set the timer for 14 minutes at MAX temperature. Press the START/STOP button to allow the unit to preheat.
2. In a large-sized bowl, toss the eggplant sliced with oil until coated well.
3. Once the unit beeps and is ready to cook, arrange the eggplants on the grill grate. Secure the grill hood and cook for 8 to 12 minutes until slightly charred on both sides.
4. Once 12 minutes are up, place one slice of mozzarella and tomato on each slice of eggplant. Allow the vegetable to cook again until the cheese melts.
5. Once the cooking cycle is over, transfer the eggplants to a serving plate to form stacks. Season with salt and pepper, and top generously with cilantro leaves. Serve while still warm.

SWEET CORN CHOWDER

PREP TIME: 15 MINS | COOK TIME: 50 MINS | SERVES 4

INGREDIENTS:

- Salt (as required)
- 1/2 tsp. Black pepper (and as required)
- 2 tbsp. Canola oil
- 3 tbsp. Butter (unsalted)
- 2 1/2 cup Vegetable broth
- 1 1/2 cup Milk
- 2 cup half and half
- 1 1/2 tsp. Fresh parsley (finely chopped)
- 4 cup Potatoes (diced)
- 1 Onion (finely chopped)
- 4 Corn ears (shucked)

DIRECTIONS:

1. Place the grill grate inside the Foodi Grill and secure the hood. Set the timer for 12 minutes at MAX temperature. Press the START/STOP button to allow the unit to heat.
2. Next, brush the corn with 1/2 tbsp. oil and season lightly with pepper and salt.
3. Once the unit beeps and is ready to cook, arrange the corn ears on the grill grate and close the grill hood. Let the corn cook for 6 minutes.
4. Once 6 minutes have passed, open the hood and turn the corn ears. Cook for the remainder of the time.
5. Once the cooking cycle is over, transfer the corn to a serving plate and allow it to cool. After the corn ears have cooled, detach the kernels from the cobs.
6. Purée one cup of kernels in a food processor until smooth consistency forms.
7. Melt the butter in a large-sized pot, and sauté the onion for 5 to 7 minutes. Next, add the broth, milk, and potatoes. Cook the potatoes for 12 minutes or until tender. Season with pepper and salt.
8. Add the corn purée mixture and remaining kernels to the potatoes and combine the half-and-half. Cook the contents for 15 to 20 minutes, or until the potatoes are cooked well. Make sure to stir the ingredients occasionally.
9. Use a potato masher to mash some of the potatoes. Add parsley, salt, and pepper to finish.

GRILLED CAULIFLOWER & BACON

PREP TIME: 10 MINS | COOK TIME: 15 MINS | SERVES 2

INGREDIENTS:

- Sea salt (as required)
- Black pepper (as required)
- 1/2 tsp. Garlic powder
- 1/2 tsp. Onion powder
- 1/2 tsp. Paprika
- 1/4 cup Canola oil

- 1 cup Cheddar (grated)
- 1 Cauliflower head (leaves removed, stemmed)
- 2 tbsp. Fresh chives (finely chopped)
- 4 Bacon slices (cooked, chopped)
- Ranch dressing (for garnish)

DIRECTIONS:

1. Start by cutting the cauliflower to form two 2-inch steaks. Reserve the remaining cauliflower for later.
2. Place the grill grate inside the Foodi Grill and choose the 'GRILL' option. Set the timer to 15 minutes at MAX temperature. Press the START/STOP button to allow the unit to preheat.
3. Whisk the garlic powder, onion powder, oil, and paprika in a small bowl. Add salt and pepper as required. Brush the cauliflower steaks with the oil mixture on all sides.
4. Once the unit beeps and is ready to cook, arrange the cauliflower on the grill grate and cook for 10 minutes.
5. Once 10 minutes have passed, open the grill hood to turn the steaks over. Top the steaks with cheese and secure the hood yet again. Cook for 5 minutes or until the cheese melts.
6. When the cooking cycle is complete, transfer the cauliflower steaks to serving plates and top with bacon, chives, and Ranch dressing.

ZUCCHINI & PEPPER PIZZA

PREP TIME: 10 MINS | COOK TIME: 10 MINS | SERVES 2

INGREDIENTS:

- Salt (as required)
- Black pepper (as required)
- 1 tsp. Garlic powder
- 1 tbsp. Canola oil (equally divided)
- 2 tbsp. All-purpose flour (and as required)
- 1/2 cup Pizza sauce

- 1 cup Mozzarella (shredded)
- 1/2 Zucchini (thinly sliced)
- 1/2 Onion (thinly sliced)
- 1/2 Red bell pepper (de-seeded, thinly sliced)
- 8 Oz. Pizza dough (ready made)

DIRECTIONS:

1. Place the grill grate inside the Foodi Grill and secure the hood. Choose the 'GRILL' option and set the timer for 7 minutes at MAX temperature. Press the START/STOP button to start the preheating process.
2. Dust a clean work surface with flour, place the pizza dough on it, and roll it into a 9-inch circle. Make sure to keep the dough's thickness even throughout.
3. Brush the rolled out pizza dough with oil, and poke the dough with a fork 4 or 5 times to prevent air pockets while cooking.
4. Once the unit beeps and is ready to cook, place the dough on the grill grate and cook for 4 minutes.
5. Once 4 minutes have passed, open the hood to turn the dough and then spread a generous layer of pizza sauce on it. Next, sprinkle the cheese and top with onion, bell pepper, and zucchini.
6. Secure the hood and cook the pizza for 2 to 3 minutes or until the cheese melts and the vegetables begin to crisp.
7. When the cooking cycle is complete, transfer the pizza to a serving plate, season with salt and pepper (optional), and serve.

VEGGIE PARMESAN SALAD

PREP TIME: 10 MINS | COOK TIME: 15 MINS | SERVES 4

INGREDIENTS:

- 1/4 tsp. Sea salt (fine)
- Black pepper (freshly ground, as required)
- 1 pinch Red pepper flakes
- 1 tbsp. Canola oil
- 2 tbsp. Olive oil (extra virgin)
- 1 tsp. Honey
- 1 tsp. Dijon mustard
- 1 tsp. Blue cheese dressing
- 1 tbsp. Lemon juice (freshly squeezed)
- 2 tbsp. Parmesan (shredded or grated)
- 1 Garlic clove (minced)
- 1/2 Onion (roughly sliced)
- 4 cups Arugula (shred by hand)
- 2 Broccoli heads (cut into florets)

DIRECTIONS:

1. Place the grill grate inside the Foodi Grill. Choose the 'GRILL' option and set the timer for 12 minutes at MAX temperature. Press the START/STOP to allow the unit to preheat.
2. Add the broccoli florets, sliced onions, and canola oil in a large-sized bowl and toss.
3. Once the unit beeps and is ready to cook, arrange the broccoli (and onions) on the grill grate and cook for 9 to 12 minutes or until the vegetables are slightly charred.
4. Next, whisk the lemon juice, olive oil, red pepper flakes, mustard, honey, blue cheese dressing, salt, and pepper in a medium-sized bowl until the ingredients are well combined. Set the sauce aside.
5. Once the grill's cooking cycle is complete, transfer the vegetables to a serving plate and add a side of arugula. Drizzle the salad and the broccoli with the dressing and parmesan cheese to serve.

SUMMER SQUASH SALAD

PREP TIME: 10 MINS | COOK TIME: 20 MINS | SERVES 4

INGREDIENTS:

- Sea salt (as required)
- Black pepper (as required)
- 2 tsp. Lemon juice (freshly juiced)
- 3 tbsp. Canola oil (divided as per directions)
- 1 Zucchini (cut lengthwise with 1/4-inch thickness)
- 1/2 Onion (sliced)
- 1 Summer squash (cut lengthwise with 1/4-inch thickness)
- 2 Portobello mushrooms (caps only, with grills removed)

DIRECTIONS:

1. Place the grill grate inside the Ninja Foodi Grill and secure the hood. Choose the 'GRILL' option and set the timer for 25 minutes at MAX temperature. Press the START/STOP button to allow the unit to preheat.
2. Toss the squash, onion, and zucchini with 2 tbsp. of oil in a large-sized bowl until the vegetables are well coated.
3. Once the unit beeps and is ready to cook, arrange the squash, zucchini, and onions on the grill grate and cook for 6 minutes.
4. After 6 minutes have passed, open the grill grate to turn the squash over and cook for another 7 to 9 minutes.
5. Brush the Portobello mushrooms with 1 tbsp. of oil. Set aside for use later.
6. When the cooking cycle is complete, transfer the vegetables to an adequately-sized plate. Add the mushrooms to the grill grate and cook for the remainder of the time.
7. When the mushrooms are done cooking, transfer them to a plate to cool.
8. Next, rough chop all the grilled vegetables and add to a medium-sized bowl. Drizzle generously with lemon juice, season with salt and pepper.

CHEESY RICE STUFFED PEPPERS

PREP TIME: 15 MINS | COOK TIME: 32 MINS | SERVES 6

INGREDIENTS:

- Sea salt (as required)
- ½ tsp. Chili powder
- ¼ tsp. Coriander (ground)
- 4 Garlic cloves (minced)
- 1 Onion (finely chopped)
- 6 Red bell peppers (de-seeded, top ½-inch cut and reserved)

- 10 oz. can of Red enchilada sauce
- ½ cup Frozen corn
- ½ cup Black beans (drained, rinsed)
- ½ cup Vegetable stock
- 8 oz. Colby Jack cheese (shredded)
- 8.5 oz. Instant rice (prepared in the microwave)

DIRECTIONS:

1. Start by chopping the ½-inch reserved bell peppers and add them to a large-sized bowl. Then as the onion, instant rice (cooked), garlic, enchilada sauce, ground coriander, corn, vegetable stock, black beans, and 4 oz. of cheese to the bowl and combine well.
2. Add the cooking pot (only) to the Ninja Foodi Grill and secure the hood. Choose the 'ROAST' option and set the timer for 32 minutes at 350°F. Press the START/STOP button to allow the unit to preheat.
3. Next, spoon the rice mixture into the remaining peppers and fill them to the top.
4. When the unit beeps and is ready to cook, place the peppers inside the cooking pot and cook for 30 minutes.
5. Once 30 minutes are up, open the grill hood and generously sprinkle the remaining cheese atop the peppers. Close the hood and cook for the remainder of the time.
6. When the cooking cycle is complete, transfer the peppers to a serving plate and serve.

MINI VEGGIE BURGERS

PREP TIME: 10 MINS | COOK TIME: 8 MINS | SERVES 4

INGREDIENTS:

- Salt (as required)
- Black pepper (as required)
- 2 tbsp. Canola oil
- 2 tbsp. Balsamic vinegar
- ½ cup Microgreens
- ½ cup Pesto

- 1 Tomato (sliced)
- 8 Portobello mushrooms (gills removed, trimmed)
- 8 Slider buns

DIRECTIONS:

1. Place the grill grate inside the Foodi Grill and secure the hood. Choose the 'GRILL' option and set the timer for 8 minutes at HIGH temperature. Press the START/STOP button to allow the unit to preheat.
2. Next, brush the mushrooms with a mixture of oil and balsamic vinegar.
3. Once the unit beeps and is heated, place the mushrooms (gill-side facing down) on the grill grate and secure the hood. Grill the mushrooms for 8 minutes or until the mushrooms are tender.
4. Once the cooking cycle is complete, start preparing the sliders by layering the buns with pesto, microgreens, tomato slices, and the grilled portobello mushrooms.

PEPPER JACK TURNOVERS

PREP TIME: 10 MINS | COOK TIME: 24 MINS | SERVES 4

INGREDIENTS:

- Cooking spray
- Salt (as required)
- 2 tbsp. Olive oil (extra-virgin)
- 1 Egg (beaten well)
- 3 tbsp. All-purpose flour (reserve an additional tbsp. for dusting)

- 1/4 tsp. Red pepper flakes
- 2 cup Pepper Jack cheese
- 1 cup Ricotta
- ½ cup Parmesan (shredded)
- Zest of 1 lemon (grated or shredded)
- 1 Garlic clove (shredded)

- 1 Cauliflower head (cut to florets)
- 16 oz. Pizza dough (ready-made)

DIRECTIONS:

1. Place the crisper basket inside the Foodi Grill and choose the 'AIR CRISP' option. Set the timer for 12 minutes at 390°F and press the START/STOP button to start the preheating process.
2. Next, add the olive oil and broccoli florets to an adequately-sized bowl and toss.
3. When the unit beeps and is ready to cook, arrange the broccoli on the grill grate and cook for 6 minutes.
4. Take the ready-made pizza dough and divide it into 4 equal portions. Dust a flat work surface with all-purpose flour, and proceed to roll each pizza dough portion until 8 inches in roundness. Make sure to dust the rolling pin with some flour to avoid the dough from sticking or tearing. Once you've rolled out all 4 portions, brush a thin coat of egg around the edges.
5. After 6 minutes have passed, take the crisper basket out of the grill to give the vegetables a little shake. Place back in the grill and cook for the reminder of the time.
6. In a medium-sized bowl, add the ricotta, parmesan, garlic, lemon zest, mozzarella, red pepper flakes, salt, and pepper. Mix the ingredients until well combined.
7. Once the broccoli is done cooking, add it to the cheese mixture. Divide the cheese mixture into four portions, and spoon each portion on one side of the rolled out pizza dough. Proceed to fold the other half of the dough over the filling, and press the edges of the dough together to seal. Brush the uncooked calzones with egg on all sides.
8. Place the crisper basket inside the grill yet again and choose the 'AIR CRISP' option. Set the timer for 12 minutes at 390°F and press the START/STOP button to allow the unit to preheat.
9. Once the unit beeps and is ready to cook, place the calzones in the crisper basket (lightly greased with cooking spray) and cook for 12 minutes or until golden brown.

GRILLED SHISHITO PEPPERS

PREP TIME: 5 MINS | COOK TIME: 10 MINS | SERVES 4

INGREDIENTS:

- 1/8 tsp Sea salt (coarse)
- 1/8 tsp Black pepper (freshly ground)
- 3 cup Shishito peppers (whole)
- 2 tbsp. Canola oil

DIRECTIONS:

1. Place the grill grate inside the Foodi Grill and choose the 'GRILL' option. Set the timer for 10 minutes at MAX temperature. Press the START/STOP button to allow the unit to preheat.
2. In a medium-sized bowl, toss the peppers with oil, salt and pepper to coat them.
3. Once the unit beeps and is ready to cook, arrange the peppers on the grill grate. Remember to press down on the peppers lightly to ensure grill marks. Secure the hood and grill the peppers for 10 minutes until they're well grilled on all sides.
4. Once the cooking cycle is over, place the peppers on a serving plate. Serve hot.

GARLIC & THYME GRILLED ARTICHOKES

PREP TIME: 10 MINS | COOK TIME: 10 MINS | SERVES 4

INGREDIENTS:

- Sea salt (small pinch)
- Black pepper (freshly ground, small pinch)
- ½ cup Canola oil
- 2 thyme sprigs
- 3 Garlic cloves (minced)
- Juice of ½ lemon
- 2 Artichokes (trimmed, halved)

DIRECTIONS:

1. Place the grill grates inside the Foodi Grill and secure the hood. Set the timer for 10 minutes at MAX temperature. Press the START/STOP button to allow the unit to preheat.
2. In an adequately-sized bowl, place the garlic, oil, thyme, salt, pepper and lemon juice. Stir until the ingredients are well combined. Brush the artichoke halves with the lemon juice mixture.
3. Once the unit beeps and is ready to cook, arrange the artichoke halves on the grill grate (cut side facing down). Remember to press down on the artichokes lightly to ensure grill marks. Secure the grill hood and cook for 10 minutes and baste the artichokes with the lemon mixture at regular intervals. Once the cooking cycle is over, transfer the artichokes to a platter, and serve.

CRISPY PAPRIKA PICKLES

PREP TIME: 10 MINS | COOK TIME: 10 MINS | SERVES 4

INGREDIENTS:

- 1/8 tsp. Salt
- 1/8 tsp. Baking powder
- 1 tsp. Paprika
- 1 tsp. Garlic powder
- 3 tbsp. Beer
- 2 tbsp. Canola oil
- Water (as required)
- 1½ cup Panko bread crumbs
- 1/4 cup All-purpose flour
- 20 Dill pickle slices (rinsed)

DIRECTIONS:

1. Start by patting the dill pickle slices dry. Arrange the slices on a plate and place in the freezer.
2. In a medium-sized bowl, add the baking powder, beer, flour, salt, and water (start with 2 tbsp. and add more if required) and mix well. The batter's consistency should resemble cake batter, so be sure to add water incrementally.
3. Add the cornstarch in a separate bowl.
4. In a large-sized bowl, combine the paprika, garlic powder, and bread crumbs. Stir the mixture with a spoon until well combined.
5. Take the dill pickle out of the freezer and dredge each slice in cornstarch first, then dip in the batter. Finally, coat with the bread crumb mixture.
6. Place the crisper basket inside the Foodi Grill choose the 'AIR CRISP' option. Set the timer for 10 minutes at 360°F. Press the START/STOP to begin preheating.
7. Once the unit beeps and is ready to cook, arrange the dill pickle slices in the basket and lightly brush with oil. Secure the grill hood and cook for 5 minutes.
8. Once 5 minutes are up, take the crisper basket out and give it a slight shake. Gently brush the pickle slices with oil again, and place back inside the grill to cook for the remaining time.
9. Once the cooking cycle is over, transfer the dill pickle slices to a serving plate and serve straight away.

LEMONY GREEN BEANS

PREP TIME: 5 MINS | COOK TIME: 10 MINS | SERVES 4

INGREDIENTS:

- Sea salt (coarse, as required)
- Black pepper (as required)
- 2 tbsp. Vegetable oil
- Juice of 1 lemon (freshly squeezed)
- 1 lb. Green beans (trimmed)

DIRECTIONS:

1. Place the grill grate inside the Ninja Foodi Grill and secure the hood. Choose the 'GRILL' option and set the timer for 10 minutes at MAX temperature. Press the START/STOP button to allow the unit to preheat.
2. In an adequately-sized bowl, toss the green beans with oil to coat them.
3. When the unit beeps and is ready to cook, arrange the green beans on the grill grate and grill for 10 minutes. Remember to stir the beans gently with a wooden spoon at regular intervals.
4. When the cooking cycle is complete, transfer the green beans to a platter. Sprinkle lemon juice, sea salt, black pepper, and serve.

BACON & BRUSSELS SPROUT BOMBS

PREP TIME: 10 MINS | COOK TIME: 12 MINS | SERVES 4

INGREDIENTS:

- 1 tsp. Sea salt
- ½ tsp. White pepper
- 2 tbsp. Olive oil (extra virgin)
- 1 lb. Brussel sprouts (trimmed, halved)
- 6 Bacon slices (diced)

DIRECTIONS:

1. Place the crisper basket inside the Foodi Grill and secure the hood. Choose the 'AIR CRISP' option and set the timer for 12 minutes at 390°F. Press the START/STOP button to allow the unit to preheat.
2. In a large-sized bowl, toss the brussel sprouts with olive oil, white pepper, salt, and bacon.
3. Once the unit beeps and is ready to cook, arrange the brussel sprouts in the basket and secure the hood. Proceed to cook the brussel sprouts for 10 minutes.
4. Once 6 minutes have passed, take the crisper basket out to give it a slight shake. Place it back inside the unit and cook for the remainder of the time.
5. When the cooking cycle is complete, check the brussel sprouts for crispness. If more time is required, cook for an additional 2 minutes and then serve.

GRILLED SOY BROCCOLI

PREP TIME: 10 MINS | COOK TIME: 10 MINS | SERVES 4

INGREDIENTS:

- 2 tbsp. Canola oil
- 4 tbsp. Soy sauce
- 4 tbsp. Balsamic vinegar
- 2 tsp. Maple syrup
- 2 Broccoli heads (cut into florets)
- Red pepper flakes (for garnish)

DIRECTIONS:

1. Place the grill grate inside the Ninja Foodi Grill and choose the 'GRILL' option. Set the timer for 10 minutes at MAX temperature. Press the START/STOPto allow the unit to preheat.
2. In a large-sized bowl, add the balsamic vinegar, soy sauce, oil, and maple syrup. Stir until all the ingredients are well combined. Add the broccoli to the sauce mixture and toss to coat evenly.
3. Once the unit beeps and is ready to cook, arrange the broccoli on the grill grate and secure the hood. Let the cooking commence, and grill the broccoli for 10 minutes.
4. After the cooking cycle is complete, transfer the broccoli florets to a platter and garnish with red pepper flakes.

CHARRED SQUASH WITH FETA

PREP TIME: 15 MINS | COOK TIME: 30 MINS | SERVES 4

INGREDIENTS:

- Sea salt (as required)
- Red pepper flakes (as required)
- ½ cup Vegetable oil (besides 3 tbsp. oil for coating vegetables)
- ¼ White wine vinegar
- 1 Onion (cut into wedges)
- 2 Summer squash (cut lengthwise to 1/4-inch slices)
- 1 Garlic clove (finely chopped)
- 8 oz. Feta cheese (crumbled)

DIRECTIONS:

1. Place the grill grate inside the Foodi grill and choose the 'GRILL' option. Set the timer for 15 minutes at MAX temperature. Press the START/STOP to start the preheating process.
2. In a small-sized bowl, whisk the vinegar, ½ cup oil, and garlic. Set aside for later use.
3. Next, toss the onion and squash in a large-sized bowl with 3 tbsp of oil until evenly coated. Season the vegetables with salt and red pepper flakes.
4. When the unit beeps, arrange the onions and squash on the grill grate and cook for 6 minutes.
5. Once 6 minutes are up, open the grill hood and turn the squash. Proceed to cook the vegetables for the remainder of the time.
6. When the cooking cycle is finished, transfer the vegetables to a platter and sprinkle generously with crumbled feta cheese. Drizzle with vinaigrette and serve after 5 minutes.

GOLDEN MAPLE CARROTS

PREP TIME: 10 MINS | COOK TIME: 10 MINS | SERVES 4

INGREDIENTS:

- 1 tbsp. Canola oil
- 1/8 tsp. Sea salt
- 1/2 tsp. Black pepper (freshly ground)
- 1/8 tsp Red pepper flakes
- 2 tbsp Butter (unsalted, melted)
- 1/4 cup Brown sugar (melted)
- 1/4 cup Maple syrup
- 6 Carrots (peeled, halved lengthwise)

DIRECTIONS:

1. Place the grill grate inside the Foodi Grill. Choose the 'GRILL' option and set the timer for 10 minutes at MAX temperature. Secure the hood and press the START/STOP to start the preheating process.
2. In a large-sized bowl, toss the carrots with oil until well coated.
3. When the unit beeps, arrange the carrots on the grill grate (in the center) and cook for 5 minutes.
4. Next, take a small-sized bowl and whisk the brown sugar, butter, maple syrup, red pepper flakes, salt, and black pepper until well combined.
5. Once 5 minutes are up, open the grill hood to baste the carrots with the maple mixture. Then turn the carrots using tongs. Proceed to baste the other side of the carrots as well. Secure the hood and cook for the remainder of the time.
6. Once the cooking cycle is complete, transfer the carrots to a platter and serve.

CRISP BABY POTATOES

PREP TIME: 20 MINS | COOK TIME: 10 MINS | SERVES 4

INGREDIENTS:

- ½ tsp. Sea salt
- ½ tsp Black pepper (freshly ground)
- 2 tbsp. Olive oil
- 1 tsp. Rosemary (dried)
- ½ tsp. Onion Powder
- ¼ tsp. Garlic powder
- ¼ cup Onion flakes (dried)
- 2 lbs. Baby red potatoes (quartered)

DIRECTIONS:

1. Place the crisper basket inside the Foodi Grill and secure the hood. Choose the 'AIR CRISP' option and set the timer for 20 minutes at 390°F. Press the START/STOP to start the preheating process.
2. Add all the ingredients to a large-sized bowl and toss until the potatoes are coated well.
3. Once the unit beeps, arrange the potatoes in the basket and cook for 10 minutes.
4. After 10 minutes are up, open the grill hood and take the basket out to give it a slight shake. Place the crisper basket back in and cook for the remainder of the time.
5. Once the cooking cycle is complete, check the potatoes to see if they're done. If they're not crisp enough, cook for an additional 5 minutes and then serve.

CRUNCHY FRENCH FRIES

PREP TIME: 15 MINS | COOK TIME: 25 MINS | SERVES 4

INGREDIENTS:

- Salt (as required)
- 3 tbsp. Canola oil
- 1 lb. Idaho potatoes (cut into 2-inch strips)

DIRECTIONS:

1. Soak the potatoes in a large-sized bowl filled with cold water for 30 minutes, then drain and pat dry with a paper towel.
2. Place the crisper basket inside the Foodi Grill and choose the 'AIR CRISP' option. Set the timer for 25 minutes at 390°F and press the START/STOP to allow the unit to preheat.
3. Next, toss the dried potatoes with oil in a large-sized bowl.
4. When the unit beeps, add the potato strips to the basket. Secure the grill hood and cook for 10 minutes.
5. Once 10 minutes have passed, take the crisper basket out and give it a slight shake. Place back inside the unit and cook for the remainder of the time.
6. Once the timer runs out, check to see if the fries are crisp. If not, cook for an additional 5 minutes.
7. When the fries are done, transfer them to a platter, and sprinkle salt. Serve with your preferred sauce.

AIR FRIED SWEET POTATOES

PREP TIME: 5 MINS | COOK TIME: 35 MINS | SERVES 4

INGREDIENTS:

- 4 Sweet potatoes
- 2 tbsp. Olive oil
- ½ tsp. Salt (optional)

DIRECTIONS:

1. Rub the sweet potatoes with olive oil and salt with your hands.
2. Place the air fryer basket in the Foodi grill and set the timer for 35 minutes at 200°F. Press the START/STOP button to start preheating.
3. Once the unit beeps, place the oiled sweet potatoes in the basket and secure the hood. Proceed to cook the potatoes for 30 minutes.
4. Once 30 minutes are up, check to see if the sweet potatoes are cooked through. If not, cook for an additional 3 to 5 minutes.
5. After the sweet potatoes are done, transfer them to a cutting board to slice. Place the sliced potatoes on a platter, top with butter and serve.

COURGETTE CRISPS

PREP TIME: 10 MINS | COOK TIME: 30 MINS | SERVES 4

INGREDIENTS:

- Salt (as required)
- Black pepper (as required)
- 1 tbsp. Olive oil
- ½ tsp. Smoked paprika
- 1 Courgette (cut into thin slices)

DIRECTIONS:

1. Place the crisper basket inside the Foodi grill and choose the 'AIR FRY' option. Set the timer for 20 minutes at 338°F. Press the START/STOP button to start preheating.
2. Slice the courgette into thin slices and place on a paper towel to absorb excess moisture.
3. Mix all the ingredients in a large-sized bowl and make sure all the courgette slices are coated well.
4. When the unit beeps and is ready to cook, add the courgette slices to the basket. Make sure to spread the slices out even through the basket. Secure the grill hood and let the courgette cook.
5. Once the cooking cycle is over, transfer the courgette crisps to a platter and allow them to cool a bit. Serve when you're ready and store in an airtight container.

PIZZA ROLLS

PREP TIME: 5 MINS | COOK TIME: 25 MINS | SERVES 4

INGREDIENTS:

- Salt (as required)
- Black pepper (as required)
- 1 tsp. Oregano
- 1 tbsp. Olive oil
- 5.95 oz. Mozzarella (shredded)
- 7 oz. Tomato passata
- 5 Bacon slices
- 1 pack of Pizza dough (ready-made)

DIRECTIONS:

1. In a large-sized bowl, combine the oregano, oil, salt, pepper, and tomato passata and mix until well combined.
2. Place the cooking pot inside the Foodi Grill and set the timer for 10 minutes at 338°F. Press the START/STOP button to allow the unit to preheat.
3. Lightly dust a flat work surface with flour and roll out the pizza dough to your choice of thickness and size. Spread tomato sauce on the surface of the dough generously with a spoon, leaving a 1/2-inch gap from the edge.
4. Next, sprinkle half of the grated mozzarella cheese on the dough and top with bacon slices. Top the bacon with the remaining mozzarella cheese.
5. Rotate the dough to form a tight roll while making sure the ingredients don't spill out. Brush the edges of the dough with water and press them together to seal the roll. Cut the pizza roll into slices measuring 0.79 inches each.
6. Once the unit beeps, open the grill hood to line the crisper basket with parchment paper. Arrange as many pizza rolls as you can, secure the hood, and let the rolls cook for 10 minutes.
7. Transfer the cooked pizza rolls to a cutting board, and set the unit to the above specific settings for the next batch. When the Foodi Grill is ready, place the second batch of pizza rolls and cook for 10 minutes.
8. Once all the pizza rolls are ready, serve them with the garnish of choice of sour cream with chives.

DESSERTS

ROLLED APPLE PIE

PREP TIME: 15 MINS | COOK TIME: 40 MINS | SERVES 4

INGREDIENTS:

- 2 tbsp. Breadcrumbs
- ¼ tsp. Allspice
- ¼ tsp. Nutmeg
- 1 tbsp. Lemon juice (freshly squeezed)
- ½ cup Raisins
- 4 Apples (peeled, grated)
- 9.65 oz. Puff pastry dough (ready-made)
- 1 Egg (for egg wash)

DIRECTIONS:

1. Add the grated apples to a sieve and add lemon juice on top. Squeeze the apples to rid them of excess juice.
2. Transfer the apples to a large-sized bowl, and add the cinnamon, nutmeg, raisins, and sugar. Mix the ingredients until well combined.
3. Place the cooking pot inside the Foodi Grill and choose the 'BAKE' option. Set the timer for 25 minutes at 338°F and press the START/STOP button to allow the unit to preheat.
4. Lightly dust a flat work surface with flour and proceed to roll out the pastry dough. Sprinkle the center of the dough with breadcrumbs to absorb excess moisture from apples while baking. Spoon the apple mixture on top of the breadcrumbs. Next, cut the sides of the pastry into 0.39-inch strips. Starting from the top, fold a strip from the right side of the pastry at a 45° angle over the apple filling. Then do the same with the top strip from the left. Repeat this process until all the pastry strips are plaited and the apple filling is covered. Tuck any strips sticking out underneath the strudel for a neat appearance.
5. Once the unit beeps, line the cooking pot with parchment paper and place the strudel in the cooking pot (diagonally for a proper fit). Secure the lid and allow the strudel to cook for 10 minutes.
6. Beat 1 egg in a small-sized bowl to prepare the egg wash. Once 10 minutes are up, lightly brush the strudel with the egg wash and secure the hood to continue cooking for the remainder of the time.
7. Transfer the strudel to a platter once it's done cooking and wait 5 to 10 minutes for it to cool. Serve the strudel while it's warm with vanilla ice cream.

GINGERBREAD CAKE

PREP TIME: 5 MINS | COOK TIME: 35 MINS | SERVES 8

INGREDIENTS:

- Cooking spray
- 2 tbsp. Cocoa powder
- ½ tsp. Ginger powder
- ¼ tsp. Cinnamon
- ¼ tsp. Nutmeg
- 1 tsp. Allspice
- 1 tsp. Baking powder
- 1 tsp. Vanilla extract
- 2 3/4 cups Plain flour
- 3/4 cup Caster Sugar
- 3.5 oz. Canola oil
- 3.5 oz. Whole milk
- 3 Eggs

DIRECTIONS:

1. In a large-sized bowl, add all the dry ingredients and the eggs, milk, and oil. Whisk the ingredients until well combined.
2. Place the cooking pot inside the Foodi Grill and choose the 'BAKE' option. Set the timer for 30 minutes at 338°F. Press the START/STOP button to start the preheating process.
3. When the unit beeps and is ready to cook, open the grill hood and grease the cooking pot with the cooking spray lightly.
4. Pour the cake mixture into the cooking pot and secure the lid. Allow the cake to bake for 30 minutes.
5. Once 30 minutes have passed, check to see if the cake is completely cooked by inserting a skewer in its center. If the skewer comes out clean, remove the cooking pot from the unit with oven mitts.
6. Serve the cake warm or cold.

LIGHT CHOCOLATE SOUFFLÉ

PREP TIME: 15 MINS | COOK TIME: 30 MINS | SERVES 2

INGREDIENTS:

- 1 pinch of Salt
- ½ tsp. Vanilla extract
- 1/2 cup Butter
- 1/2 cup Caster sugar
- 2 Eggs (yolks & whites separated)
- ¼ cup Plain flour
- ¾ cup Chocolate (Chopped)
- Whipped cream (to serve with)

DIRECTIONS:

1. Start by preparing the ramekin by greasing their insides and lightly coat with sugar by moving it around in the ramekins. Discard the excess sugar.
2. Add the butter and chocolate to a microwave-safe bowl and melt using 30 seconds periods. Make sure to stir after microwaving each time until the ingredients are melted and well combined.
3. Whisk the egg whites in a medium-sized bowl using a beater until soft peaks form.
4. Place the crisper basket inside the Foodi Grill and choose the 'AIR FRY' option. Set the timer for 25 minutes at 375° F. Press the START/STOP button to start preheating.
5. In an adequately-sized bowl, add the sugar, egg yolks, vanilla extract, and whisk. While whisking vigorously, add the chocolate-butter mixture slowly. Continue to whisk until the ingredients are well combined.
6. Next, stir in the flour and whisk well to avoid lumps.
7. Fold in 1/3 of the egg whites gently into the souffle batter. Make sure not to blend in too energetically to avoid deflating the mixture.
8. Transfer the souffle batter to the ramekins and leave at least 0.70 inches of room at the top for the souffle to rise without spilling over.
9. When the unit beeps, place the ramekins inside the basket and secure the hood. Allow the souffle to cook for 13 minutes.
10. When the cooking cycle is complete, open the grill hood and allow the souffles to cool a bit. Transfer the ramekins from the grill unit with the help of oven mitts or tongs to serving plates.
11. Top the souffles with whipped cream and serve immediately.

RUM PINEAPPLE SUNDAES

PREP TIME: 15 MINS | COOK TIME: 8 MINS | SERVES 6

INGREDIENTS:

- 1 Pineapple (cored, sliced)
- ½ cup Dark rum
- ½ cup Brown sugar (packed)
- 1 tsp. Allspice (besides some for garnishing)
- Vanilla ice cream (to serve with)

DIRECTIONS:

1. In a large-sized bowl, add the sugar, allspice, and rum. Mix until the ingredients combine. Next, add the pineapple slices to the rum mixture and coat well. Let the pineapple soak in the mixture for 10 minutes (5 minutes per side)
2. Place the grill grate inside the Ninja Foodi Grill and choose the 'GRILL' option. Set the timer for 8 minutes at MAX temperature. Press the START/STOP button to start preheating.
3. Strain the pineapple slices from the rum mixture.
4. When the unit beeps, arrange the pineapple slices (in a single layer) on the grill grate and secure the hood. Gently press down on the slices to ensure grill marks. Secure the hood and cook for 8 minutes. Once the first batch of pineapples is done, repeat the process with the above-stated settings for the next batch(es).
5. When all the pineapple slices are done, transfer them to serving plates and serve with a side of vanilla ice cream.

GLAZED DONUTS

PREP TIME: 20 MINS | COOK TIME: 60 MINS | SERVES 12

INGREDIENTS:

For Donuts
- 1 Egg
- ½ tsp. Salt
- 2 ½ tbsp. Fresh yeast
- 1/4 cup Caster sugar

- 3 ½ cups White flour
- 1/4 cup Butter (melted)
- 1 cup Milk (lukewarm)

For the Glaze
- 3/4 cup Butter
- 1 cup Icing sugar
- 2 tsp. Vanilla extract
- ¼ tsp. Maple syrup (optional)

DIRECTIONS:

1. Add the milk, sugar, and yeast (crumbled) to the bowl of a stand mixer (fitted with the dough hook). Let the mixture sit until foam forms (to ensure the yeast is activated).
2. Next, add salt, melted butter, egg, and flour to the yeast mixture. Start the mixer and combine the ingredients on a low setting. Allow the mixer to work for 5 minutes or until the dough is smooth and elastic.
3. Detach the mixer, and cover the bowl with cling film. Set the bowl in a warm place to allow the dough to rise. The dough will be ready once you make a dent with your finger, and it remains.
4. Place the dough onto a flat work surface lightly dusted with flour and punch it gently. Roll the dough out to a 0.79-inch thickness with the help of a rolling pin. Use a donut cutter to form the donuts.
5. Move the donuts to a sheet of parchment paper and cover lightly with cling film. Allow the donuts to rise for 30 minutes.
6. Prepare the donut glaze by melting butter in a medium-sized saucepan. Then proceed to add the icing sugar, vanilla extract, maple syrup, and cook the mixture until smooth consistency forms. Remove the saucepan from the heat.
7. Place the crisper basket inside the Foodi Grill and choose the 'AIR FRY' option. Set the timer for 4 minutes at 374°F. Press the START/STOP button to start preheating.
8. When the unit beeps, arrange the donuts (in a single layer) on the crisper basket and cook for 4 minutes. Transfer the donuts to a wire rack and repeat the process with the above-stated settings for the next batch(es).
9. Dip the donuts into the glaze mixture while hot (with the help of forks) and transfer back to the wire rack (for the excess glaze to drip off). Wait until the glaze hardens, and then serve.

PEANUT BANANA PUDDING

PREP TIME: 10 MINS | COOK TIME: 6 MINS | SERVES 4

INGREDIENTS:

- 1 cup Mini marshmallows
- ½ cup Chocolate chips
- ½ cup Peanut butter chips
- 4 Bananas (ripe)
- 1 pinch of Salt

DIRECTIONS:

1. Place the grill grate inside the Foodi grill and secure the hood. Choose the 'GRILL' option and set the timer for 6 minutes at MEDIUM temperature. Press the START/STOP button to start the preheating.
2. Next, slice the bananas in half lengthwise without peeling them. Make sure not to slice the whole way through. Pull the peels apart gently using both hands. Then, stuff the bananas with mini marshmallows, chocolate chips, and peanut butter chips equally. Sprinkle the bananas with salt sparsely.
3. Once the unit beeps and is ready to cook, arrange the stuffed bananas on the grill grate and secure the grill hood. Allow the banana boats to cook for 4 to 6 minutes or until the chocolate chips and marshmallows have melted and serve.

GRILLED BOURBON PEACHES

PREP TIME: 10 MINS | COOK TIME: 12 MINS | SERVES 4

INGREDIENTS:

- ¼ cup Brown Sugar
- ¼ cup Bourbon
- 4 tbsp. Butter (salted)
- ¼ cup Glazed pecans
- 4 Ripe peaches (pitted, halved)

DIRECTIONS:

1. Place the grill grate inside the Foodi grill and secure the hood. Choose the 'GRILL' option and set the timer for 12 minutes at MAX temperature. Press the START/STOP button to start preheating.
2. Next, melt butter in a medium-sized saucepan over medium flame for 5 minutes. When the butter turns brown, remove the saucepan from the heat and add the bourbon.
3. Place the saucepan over a medium flame again and add the brown sugar. Bring the mixture to a boil and allow the sugar to dissolve while stirring occasionally.
4. Transfer the bourbon sauce to a medium-sized bowl and arrange the peached (cut side facing down) in the sauce.
5. When the unit beeps and is ready to cook, arrange the peaches on the grill grate (in a single layer). Make sure to press down on the fruit gently to ensure grill marks. Secure the grill hood and cook for 12 minutes. Once 12 minutes are up, move the cooked peaches to a platter and repeat the process (with the above-stated settings) for the next batch(es).
6. When the peaches are done, transfer them to a serving plate and top with glazed pecans. Drizzle the peaches with the rest of the bourbon sauce generously and serve.

DOUBLE BERRY POUND CAKE

PREP TIME: 10 MINS | COOK TIME: 8 MINS | SERVES 4

INGREDIENTS:

- 3 tbsp. Butter (unsalted, room temperature)
- ½ cup Raspberries (fresh)
- 1 cup blueberries (fresh)
- 3 tbsp. Sugar
- 6 Pound cake slices (cut to 1-inch thickness)

DIRECTIONS:

1. Place the grill grate inside the Foodi Grill and secure the hood. Choose the 'GRILL' option and set the timer for 8 minutes at MAX temperature. Press the START/STOP button to start preheating.
2. Next, spread an even coat of butter on both sides of the cake slices.
3. When the unit beeps, arrange the pound cake slices (in a single layer) on the grill grate and secure the hood. Allow the cake to cook for 2 minutes.
4. Once two minutes have passed, turn the cake slices and cook for another 2 minutes. Repeat the process for the next batch of cake slices.
5. In a medium-sized bowl, combine the blueberries, raspberries, and sugar.
6. After the cooking cycle is complete, transfer the cake slices to a platter. Serve warm, topped with the berry mixture.

SWEET STRAWBERRY PIZZA

PREP TIME: 10 MINS | COOK TIME: 6 MINS | SERVES 4

INGREDIENTS:

- 1 tbsp. Canola oil
- 1 tbsp. Brown sugar
- 1 cup Strawberries (fresh, sliced)
- 2 tbsp. All-purpose flour (besides some for dusting)
- 8 oz. Pizza dough
- 1 cup Nutella

DIRECTIONS:

1. Place the grill grate inside the Foodi grill and choose the 'GRILL option. Set the timer for 6 minutes at MAX temperature. Press the START/STOP to start the preheating process.
2. Dust a flat work surface with the all-purpose flour and roll it to a 9-inch circle of even thickness. Work the rolled out dough with additional flour by dusting the rolling pin.
3. Next, brush the surface ½ tsp. of oil. Use a fork to poke the dough in 5 to 6 places to avoid air pockets while cooking.
4. Once the unit beeps and is ready to cook, transfer the dough to the grill grate. Secure the grill hood and cook for 3 minutes.
5. Once 3 minutes are up, open the grill hood to turn the dough. Proceed to cook for another 3 minutes.
6. In a medium-sized bowl, combine the strawberries with sugar and mix well.
7. Once the pizza dough is cooked, transfer it to a cutting board and allow it cool for 5 to 10 minutes. Top the pizza with the Nutella and evenly spread it. Next, spatter the spread with the strawberry slices generously. Cut the pizza in pieces and serve.

OLD-FASHIONED BLUEBERRY CRUMBLE

PREP TIME: 15 MINS | COOK TIME: 30 MINS | SERVES 6

INGREDIENTS:

- 1 tsp. Lemon zest (grated)
- 2 tsp. Baking powder
- ¼ tsp. Salt
- 1/8 tsp. Allspice
- 6 tbsp. Butter (unsalted)
- 1 cup Sugar (plus 2 additional tbsp.)
- 1 cup All-purpose flour (plus 2 additional tbsp.)
- ¾ cup Milk
- 4 cups Blueberries (fresh)
- Juice of 1 lemon

DIRECTIONS:

1. Mix the blueberries, 2 tbsp. sugar, 2 tbsp. flour, lemon juice, and lemon zest in a medium-sized bowl.
2. In a large-sized bowl, add 1 cup flour, baking powder, salt, and 1 cup sugar. Add the butter and stir (or mix with hands) until the mixture forms a crumbly texture. Proceed to add the milk and mix until a dough forms.
3. Choose the 'BAKE' option on the Foodi grill and set the timer for 30 minutes at 350°F, and press the START/STOP to allow the unit to preheat.
4. Pour the blueberry mixture into the Ninja All-purpose pan and spread it evenly across the pan's surface. Next, pour the batter over the blueberries gently and sprinkle the allspice on top.
5. When the unit beeps and is ready to cook, place the pan into the Foodi grill, and secure the hood. Cook for 30 minutes or until golden brown.
6. Once the cooking cycle is complete, remove the pan from the grill and let it cool for 5 minutes. Serve warm with a preferred side option like vanilla ice cream.

SWEET CINNAMON BISCUITS

PREP TIME: 15 MINS | COOK TIME: 12 MINS | SERVES 8

INGREDIENTS:

- Cooking spray
- ¼ tsp. Sea salt
- ¼ tsp. Cinnamon (ground)
- ¼ tsp. Nutmeg (ground)
- 1 tsp. Baking powder
- 2 tbsp. Sugar (granulated)
- 2 tbsp Water
- 4 tbsp. Butter (salted, cut into small pieces)
- 2/3 cup All-purpose flour (besides 2 additional tbsp. for dusting)
- 2/3 cup Whole wheat flour
- 2 cup Icing sugar

DIRECTIONS:

1. Combine the whole wheat flour, all-purpose flour, cinnamon, nutmeg, baking powder, sugar, and salt in a large-sized bowl. Next, add the butter pieces and mix them with the other ingredients using a fork until the mixture looks coarse or crumbly. Proceed to add milk into the mixture and mix until a dough forms.
2. Place the crisper basket inside the Foodi grill and secure the hood. Choose the 'AIR CRISP' option and set the timer for 12 minutes at 350°F. Press the START/STOP button to start preheating.
3. Knead the dough on a lightly dusted flat work surface until there are no lumps and the dough looks smooth and cohesive. Divide the dough into 16 equal portions and roll each piece into a ball.
4. When the unit beeps and is ready to cook, grease the crisper basket with cooking spray. Transfer 8 biscuit bites to the crisper basket and leave at least a ½-inch gap between them. Secure the hood and cook the biscuits for 12 minutes or until golden brown.
5. In a medium-sized bowl, add the sugar and water and whisk until a smooth glaze is formed.
6. Once the biscuit bites are ready, remove them from the basket and transfer to a wire rack to cool. Cover the biscuits lightly with aluminum foil. Repeat the cooking process for the remaining biscuit bites with the above-stated settings.
7. Spoon the first batch of biscuit bites with the glaze while they're still warm. Do the same for the second batch once they're ready. Serve warm, or whenever you please.

BUTTERMILK BISCUITS

PREP TIME: 15 MINS | COOK TIME: 15 MINS | SERVES 6

INGREDIENTS:

- Cooking spray
- 1/2 tsp. Sea salt
- 1/8 tsp. Sugar
- 2 ½ tsp. Baking powder
- 2/3 cup Buttermilk
- 1/3 cup Vegetable shortening
- ½ cup Yellow cornmeal

DIRECTIONS:

1. Combine the cornmeal, flour, baking powder, sugar, and salt in a large-sized bowl.
2. Add vegetable shortening to the bowl and cut it into the cornmeal mixture until coarse consistency forms. Next, add the buttermilk to the mixture and stir the ingredients until well combined.
3. Place the crisper basket inside the Ninja Foodi grill and secure the hood. Choose the 'AIR CRISP' option and set the timer for 15 minutes at 350°F. Press the START/STOP button to start the preheating.
4. Dust a flat work surface with flour and place the cornmeal dough on it. Knead the mixture until it forms a uniform cohesiveness. Roll out the dough to preferred dimensions and make sure the thickness is even throughout. Use a 2-inch biscuit-cutter to cut out the biscuits.
5. When the unit beeps and is ready to cook, grease the basket with cooking spray and arrange 8 biscuits in it. Make sure to keep ample space in between the biscuits. Secure the hood and cook the biscuits for 12 minutes or until golden brown.
6. Once the cooking cycle is complete, transfer the biscuits to a wire rack and add the next batch of biscuits to the grill. Cook the biscuits at the above-mentioned settings.
7. Serve the biscuits warm.

CRISPY CHOCO CHURROS

PREP TIME: 15 MINS | COOK TIME: 30 MINS | SERVES 8

INGREDIENTS:

- Cooking spray
- 3 Eggs (large)
- 2 tbsp. Allspice
- 1 tsp. Vanilla extract
- ½ cup Sugar (besides 1 additional tbsp.)
- 1 cup Water
- 1 cup All-purpose flour
- ¼ cup Greek yogurt
- 1 Stick of butter (unsalted, cut into 8 pieces)
- 4 oz. Dark chocolate (chopped)

DIRECTIONS:

1. Combine the butter, water, and 1 tbsp sugar in a medium-sized saucepan over medium-high heat. Stir occasionally and bring the mixture to a simmer. Next, stir quickly, as you add in the flour. Continue to cook, and stir constantly (to avoid lumps) for 3 minutes or until the mixture is thick. Remove from heat and transfer the mixture to a large-sized bowl.
2. Beat the flour mixture for 1 minute with the help of a spoon to help it cool slightly. Then add the eggs (one at a time) and vanilla extract and mix until well combined.
3. Transfer the flour mixture to a piping bag from the bowl. Allow the dough to rest at room temperature for at least 1 hour.
4. Place the crisper basket inside the Foodi grill and choose the 'AIR CRISP' option. Set the timer for 30 minutes at 375°F. Press the START/STOP button to start the preheating process.
5. In a medium-sized bowl, combine the allspice and remaining (½ cup) sugar.
6. Once the unit beeps and is ready to cook, spray the basket with a thin coat of cooking spray. Take the piping bag and pipe the churros batter directly into the basket. Make sure each churro is at least 3 inches long and pipe the churros with a ½-inch gap. Secure the hood and cook for 10 minutes.
7. Melt the chocolate in a microwave-safe bowl by cooking it for 30 second periods. Make sure to stir after each 30-second period. Continue the process until the chocolate is smooth and melted. Next, add the greek yogurt to the melted chocolate and whisk until well combined.
8. Once 10 minutes are up, transfer the cooked churros to the sugar and allspice mixture to coat them. Repeat the piping and cooking process with the above-stated settings for the remaining batches of churros.
9. Once the churros are ready, transfer them to a serving plate and drizzle with the chocolate and yogurt mixture. Serve warm.

FRIED OREOS WITH ICING

PREP TIME: 5 MINS | COOK TIME: 10 MINS | SERVES 8

INGREDIENTS:

- Cooking spray
- 1 tube of Crescent roll dough
- 8 Oreos
- 2 tbsp. White icing sugar
- 1 tbsp. Milk
- ¼ tsp. Vanilla extract

DIRECTIONS:

1. Wrap each Oreo in crescent roll dough. Make sure to trim off any excess dough to give the pastry a neat look.
2. Grease the crisper basket with cooking spray and place it in the Foodi grill. Secure the hood and set the timer for 6 minutes at 350°F. Press the START/STOP button to start the preheating process.
3. While the unit is preheating, prepare the icing by whisking the sugar, milk, and vanilla extract in a small-sized bowl. Continue to whisk until smooth consistency forms.
4. Once the unit beeps, arrange the Oreos (in a single layer) and secure the hood. Allow the dough to cook for 6 minutes. Once the cooking cycle is over, remove the fried Oreos from the grill and place them on a wire rack. Prepare the unit with the above-stated settings for the next batch and repeat the process.
5. Top the fried Oreos with icing while still warm and serve.

RICH CHOC BROWNIE

PREP TIME: 15 MINS | COOK TIME: 40 MINS | SERVES 6

INGREDIENTS:

- Nonstick cooking spray
- 2 Eggs (large)
- 1 tbsp. Vanilla extract
- 1 tbsp. Water
- ¾ tsp. Sea salt
- ½ cup Granulated sugar

- ½ cup Dark brown sugar
- ¼ cup Cocoa powder (unsweetened)
- ½ cup All-purpose flour
- 8 oz. Chocolate chips (semisweet, melted)
- 1 pinch of Cinnamon (ground)

DIRECTIONS:

1. Whisk the cocoa powder, flour, cinnamon, and salt in a medium-sized bowl.
2. In a large-sized bowl, mix the sugar, water, brown sugar, vanilla extract, and eggs until a smooth mixture forms.
3. Melt the chocolate chips using the microwave (in a microwave-safe bowl. Repeat the process for the butter in another bowl.
4. In another medium-sized bowl, add the melted butter and chocolate and mix until well combined. Then add the egg mixture to the bowl slowly and mix together. Finally, add the dry ingredients and stir until all the ingredients are blended.
5. Remove the grill grate from the Foodi unit and choose the 'BAKE' option. Set the timer for 40 minutes at 350°F and press the START/STOP button to start preheating.
6. 6. Grease the Ninja multi-purpose pan with cooking spray and pour the batter into the pan gently. Spread the batter evenly across the surface of the pan.
7. Once the unit beeps and is ready to cook, insert the pan inside the Foodi grill and secure the hood. Allow the cake to cook for 40 minutes.
8. Once the cooking cycle is complete, check to see if the cake is cooked through with a wooden skewer. Stick the skewer in the center of the cake. If the skewer comes up clean, remove the pan from the grill and allow to cool for 5 to 10 minutes. Serve warm.

GRILLED CHEESECAKE

PREP TIME: 20 MINS | COOK TIME: 45 MINS | SERVES 8

INGREDIENTS:

- 2 Eggs
- 1 tbsp. Allspice
- 8 tbsp. Butter (melted)
- 2 tbsp. Sugar
- 1 tbsp. Vanilla bean paste

- 1 ¼ cup Graham cracker crumbs
- 2 cups. Cream cheese (softened)
- 1 cup Sweetened condensed milk

DIRECTIONS:

1. In a medium-sized bowl, mix the graham cracker crumbs and butter to form the cheesecake crust. Once the ingredients are well combined, transfer the crust to an 8-inch cheesecake pan and press it into place. Place the pan in the freezer.
2. Next, mix all the other ingredients in a large-sized bowl and combine well. Once the filling is ready, pour the mixture into the pan with the crust.
3. To prepare the Foodi grill, set the timer for 35 minutes at 300°F. Press the START/STOP button to start preheating. Make sure the cooking pot is placed inside the grill.
4. Once the unit beeps and is ready to cook, place the cheesecake pan with the filling inside the cooking pot, and secure the hood. Allow the cheesecake to cook for 35 minutes.
5. Once the cooking cycle is complete, remove the pan from the grill and let it cool for 5 to 10 minutes. Then place the cheesecake pan in the refrigerator for 4 hours and serve with preferred toppings.

POMEGRANATE CREAM LAYER CAKE

PREP TIME: 15 MINS | COOK TIME: 50 MINS | SERVES 8

INGREDIENTS:

- 3 eggs
- 1 Egg yolk
- ½ tsp. Vanilla extract
- ¼ tsp. Bicarbonate of soda
- ¼ tsp. Baking powder
- 1 tsp. Lemon juice
- ½ cup Caster sugar
- 3/4 cup Plain flour
- 1/3 cup pumpkin seed oil (or avocado oil)

For Whipped cream
- 2 ¼ cup Whipping cream
- 1 tsp. Vanilla bean paste
- 1/4 cup Caster sugar

For Toppings
- 1/4 cup Fresh pomegranate seeds
- 3 Ripe Plums
- 1 pack of Meringue shells

DIRECTIONS:

1. Place the cooking pot inside the Foodi Grill and secure its hood. Choose the 'BAKE' option and set the timer for 30 minutes at 338°F. Press the START/STOP button to start the preheating. Next, grease a small-sized spring form cake tin and set aside.
2. Add the yolk, sugar, vanilla bean paste, and whole eggs to a large-sized bowl and whisk with an electric mixer for 5 to 10 minutes on high speed. Continue to whisk the batter until thick ribbons form.
3. Next, in a large-sized bowl sieve the flour, bicarb. of soda, baking powder, and salt. Add the dry ingredients to the egg batter incrementally and fold together gently until well combined.
4. Add lemon juice and pumpkin seed oil next and fold them in the batter. Make sure not to over-stir the batter to avoid deflating it.
5. Once the unit beeps, add the batter to the spring form tin and place it in the cooking pot. Secure the grill hood and cook the cake for 30 minutes.
6. When the cooking cycle is over, check if the cake is cooked through by inserting a skewer in its center. If the skewer comes out wet with batter, then cook the cake for an additional 5 minutes.
7. Once the cake is ready, remove the tin from the unit and place the cake tin on a wire rack to cool.
8. Proceed to make the whipped cream by whipping cream in a large-sized bowl with an electric mixer. Whisk the cream at medium speed and when it thickens, add the vanilla bean paste and caster sugar. Continue whisking at medium speed until soft peaks form. Set aside for later use.
9. Place the grill plate inside the Foodi grill and choose the 'GRILL' option. Set the timer for 3 minutes at HIGH temperature. Press the START/STOP button to start the preheating.
10. Cut the plums into 0.39-inch (approximately) thick slices.
11. When the unit beeps and is ready to cook, arrange the persimmon slices on the grill grate and cook for 3 minutes. When the timer runs out, transfer the persimmon slices to a plate lined with parchment paper to cool. Repeat this process until all the persimmon slices are done. Set a few slices aside to decorate the cake with and cut the rest into small chunks.
12. To assemble the cake, release it from the spring form tin and remove the base as well. You can use a palette knife to help release the cake from the tin's edges. Next, use a serrated knife to cut the cake (horizontally) into 3 equal slices. Spread a layer of the whipped cream on the base layer, and top it with crumbled pieces of the meringue shells. Add a layer of persimmon chunks and pomegranate seeds on top of the shells. Then, add the next layer of cake and repeat the filling process. Place the top layer of the cake on the second layer of filling and decorate with whipped cream, persimmon slices, and pomegranate seeds as you prefer. You can also use the leftover crumbled meringue shells for the decoration.
13. Once the cake is ready, be sure to serve it on the same day. The meringue tends to soften if left out for too long or refrigerated.

BANANA SPLITS WITH A TWIST

PREP TIME: 5 MINS | COOK TIME: 15 MINS | SERVES 2

INGREDIENTS:

For Grilled Bananas
- 2 Bananas (with peel)
- 1 tbsp. Sugar
- 1 tsp. Vanilla extract
- 2 ½ tsp Butter (room temperature)

For the topping
- 1 tsp. Coconut oil
- 2 tbsp. Walnuts (chopped)
- 1 ½ tbsp. Chocolate (chopped)
- 6 Maraschino cherries

- Vanilla ice cream (to serve)
- Whipped cream (to serve)

DIRECTIONS:

1. Slice the bananas lengthwise (from top to end). Make sure not to cut the bananas the whole way through.
2. Place the grill grate inside the Foodi Grill and choose the 'GRILL' option. Set the timer for 10 minutes at LOW temperature. Press the START/STOP button to start the preheating.
3. In a medium-sized bowl, mix the butter, vanilla extract, and sugar until it forms a smooth paste. Spread this mixture in between the cuts on the banana equally.
4. When the unit beeps and is ready to cook, open the grill hood and spray the grill grate with cooking spray. Arrange the bananas on the grill grate (on their sides) and allow them to cook for 5 minutes.
5. Once 5 minutes are up, open the grill hood and turn the bananas over with the help of silicone tongs. Secure the hood and cook for the remainder of the time.
6. To make the chocolate sauce, add the coconut oil and chopped chocolate to a microwave-safe bowl, and cook for 10 second periods. Remember to stir the sauce after each 10-second cook. Continue until the chocolate is melted and well combined with the coconut oil.
7. Arrange the bananas on a platter and open their skins a little. Top the bananas with whipped cream, walnuts, and maraschino cherries. Add a scoop or two of vanilla ice cream and drizzle with delicious chocolate sauce.

CARAMEL CRUNCH BROWNIES

PREP TIME: 5 MINS | COOK TIME: 45 MINS | SERVES 8

INGREDIENTS:

- 1 pinch of Salt
- 2 tbsp Caramel
- 3 Eggs
- 1 1/8 cup Caster sugar
- 1 1/4 cup Plain flour

- 1 cup Butter (unsalted)
- 1 cup Dark Chocolate (chopped)
- 1/3 cup Biscoff spread
- 3 tbsp Biscoff biscuits (crumbled to uneven pieces)

DIRECTIONS:

1. Place the cooking pot inside the Foodi grill and choose the 'BAKE' option. Set the timer for 35 minutes at 302°F. Press the START/STOP button to allow the unit to preheat. Spray a 7 ½ -inch foil container with cooking spray and set aside.
2. Set an adequately-sized bowl over a pot of water. Make sure the bottom of the bowl isn't touching the water.
3. Next, add the chocolate and butter to the bowl and melt the two ingredients over low heat. Once the chocolate is melted and well combined with the butter, remove the bowl from the heat.
4. Allow the chocolate-butter mixture to cool for 2 to 3 minutes. Then proceed to add the sugar and eggs and whisk for 5 minutes.
5. Fold the plain flour and 1 pinch of salt in the mixture and fold until it forms a smooth consistency.
6. Add the biscoff biscuits to the batter, and pour the batter into the foil container.
7. Finally, add small-sized dollops of biscoff spread on top of the batter and swirl with a skewer or cocktail stick.
8. Place the foil container in the cooking pot and bake the batter for 35 minutes.
9. Once the cooking cycle is over, and the cake is cooked through, remove the container with oven mitts. Drizzle the cake with caramel and crumbled biscoff biscuits. Serve warm.

CONCLUSION

Well foodi's, that's it! I hope you have enjoyed cooking and eating these recipes as much as I did creating them.

Want to make the most of the recipes in this cookbook? Shop locally-grown ingredients from your neighborhood farmer's market or small grocer! These ingredients typically come from the freshest farms around, so your recipes will always taste their very best! An added bonus? Shopping locally supports the farmers in your community while reducing environmental harms and promoting long-lasting sustainability.

Happy Cooking!